101 High-Intensity
Workouts for *Fast* Results

ACKNOWLEDGEMENTS

This publication is based on articles written by David Barr, CSCS, CISSN, Jon Finkel, Bill Geiger, MA, Jimmy Peña, MS, CSCS, David Sandler, MS, CSCS, Jim Stoppani, PhD, Mark Thorpe, Eric Velazquez and Joe Wuebben

Cover photography by iconmen.com

Photography and illustrations by: Art Brewer, Michael Darter, Kevin Horton, Ian Logan, Joaquin Palting, Robert Reiff, Ismael Roldan, Marc Royce, Brian Sanchez, Ian Spanier and Pavel Ythjall

Project editor is Joe Wuebben

Project exercise science adviser is David Barr, CSCS, CISSN

Project managing editor is Jared Evans

Project copy editor is Kristina Haar

Project design by Michael Touna

Photo assistants are Amina Cruz, Yvonne Mejia

Editorial assistant is Nune Gazdhyan

Founding chairman is Joe Weider. Chairman and CEO of American Media, Inc., is David Pecker

This book is available in quantity at special discounts for your group or organization. For further information, contact:

Triumph Books
542 South Dearborn Street
Suite 750
Chicago, Illinois 60605
(312) 939-3330
Fax (312) 663-3557
www.triumphbooks.com

ISBN: 978-1-60078-338-8

Printed in USA

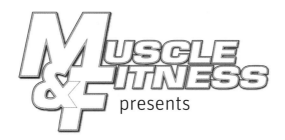

MUSCLE & FITNESS
presents

101 High-Intensity
Workouts for *Fast* Results

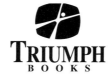

TRIUMPH
BOOKS

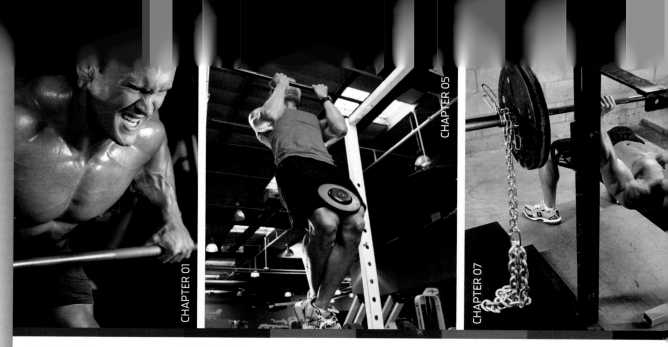

CHAPTER 01

CHAPTER 05

CHAPTER 07

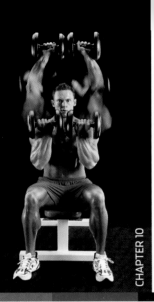

CHAPTER 10

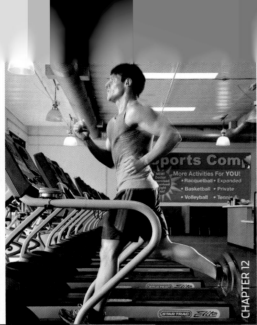

CHAPTER 12

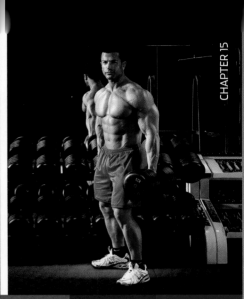

CHAPTER 15

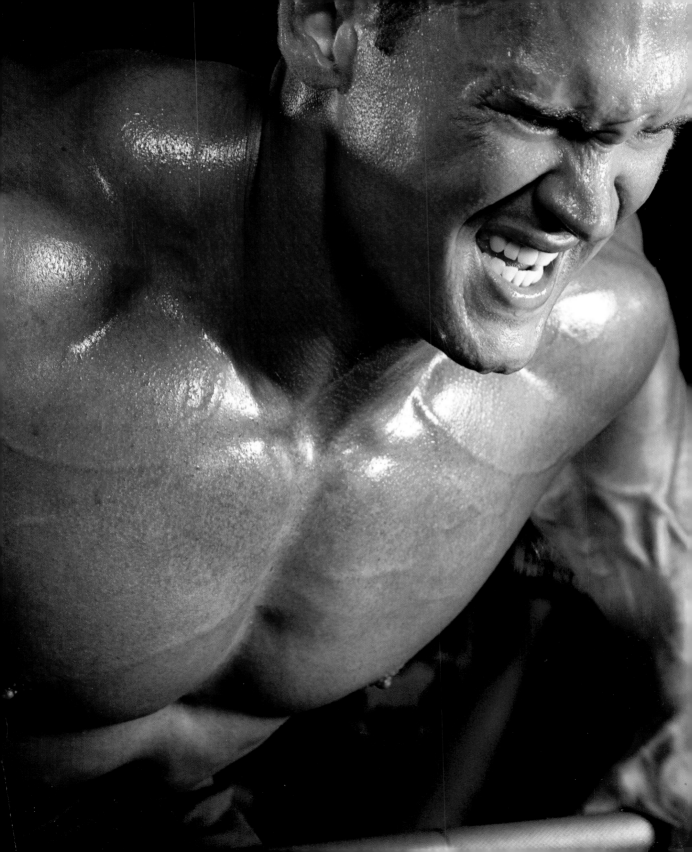

SIX KEYS TO
INTENSITY

GO BEYOND BASIC SET-AND-REP SCHEMES WITH THESE TIPS THAT WILL VOLUMIZE YOUR WORKOUT AND YOUR PHYSIQUE

To some, working out is simply about numbers. Three sets of eight. Four sets of 10. Rest one minute between sets. Do 20 total sets. But beneath every tangible number and finite measurement used to define the amount of work you've done, there's the enigmatic — albeit ever-important — variable known as intensity. In fact, this might be the most crucial training variable of all.

Intensity isn't a number. It can't be written down in a training log nearly as succinctly as, say, a tally of sets and reps you do for an exercise. And a set of 50 reps isn't necessarily more intense than a set of six. Bottom line: Where training for gains in muscle size is concerned, intensity equals muscle failure.

If your muscles fatigue to the point that you can't do another rep (aka "failure"), that's an intense set. Stopping short of failure? Not as intense. Yet intensity goes far beyond just one set — each set affects the next set, every workout affects the next workout, every week affects the next week, and so on. How you manage your intensity from set to set and workout to workout goes a long way in dictating the effectiveness of your program. That said, there's a certain hierarchy to training intensity, and the best way to articulate it is to start small (with a single rep) and pull the layers back until you see the big picture. Hence, the following six levels of intensity.

1 INTENSITY OF A REP

To ensure adequate intensity in a set, and subsequently in a workout, you first need to make sure that each and every rep is performed in an intense manner. Of course, the first few reps of a 20-rep set (in which you would use a relatively light weight) feel much different than those of a six-rep set — with the heavier weight, the reps feel difficult right away, whereas the first several reps with the lighter weight feel much easier. Yet the amount of weight you use and how many reps you plan to do in that set shouldn't affect each individual rep.

The first key to maximizing intensity at this level is to concentrate on the muscle group you're working, whether you're at the beginning or the end of a high-rep set and regardless of whether the weight feels heavy or light. This is what bodybuilders typically refer to as the "mind-muscle connection."

Second, make sure you emphasize the eccentric, or negative, portion of each rep just as much as the positive, or concentric, portion. Don't let the weight simply drop on every rep; rather, control the negative so it takes at least two seconds to lower the weight. Since it's possible to produce greater force during eccentric contractions than during concentric muscle actions, eccentric activity may be more important in producing muscle strength and size. Therefore, it's critical to control the weight's return or descent; don't just let it fall back down. Oftentimes, the negative is overlooked in high-rep sets, as well as when training heavy. Making a habit of both of these practices — concentrating on the working muscles and controlling the negative — ensures adequate intensity on each and every rep.

Third, consider the point of peak contraction (the top of the repetition where you squeeze the muscle for a moment or two before continuing through the rep). This squeezing creates more work for the muscle, driving more blood flow (aka "the pump"), which temporarily increases the muscle's size by placing a stretch on it. This stretch initiates biochemical pathways that signal the muscle to grow.

2 INTENSITY OF A SET

As mentioned earlier, how much weight you use for a given set doesn't define intensity; a set of 20 reps using 100 pounds can be just as intense as a set of five reps with 200 pounds. The measure of intensity for a set is whether it's taken to failure (the one exception being a set taken *past* failure, which we'll discuss shortly).

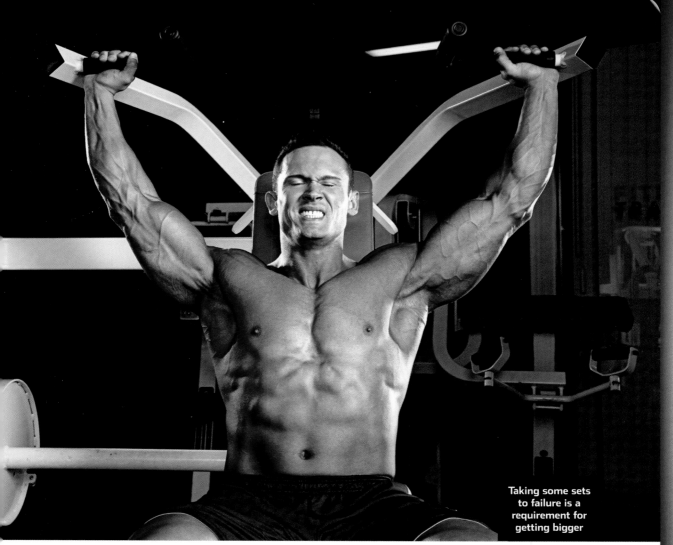

Taking some sets to failure is a requirement for getting bigger

Training to failure is defined by being physically unable to perform one more rep in a given set on your own as a result of temporary muscle fatigue. This can occur by attempting one more rep and not being able to complete it — for example, a set in which you can get the 10th rep only halfway up is officially a set of nine reps to failure. However, failing on a set can also mean that the last rep was so difficult (you barely completed the rep) that you know for certain you couldn't complete another and therefore didn't try to continue the set. On the flip side, a set of 10 reps in which you could've done a few more was not taken to failure. Naturally, a set taken to failure is more intense than a set stopped short of failure, regardless of how much weight you used.

Occasionally taking sets to failure is a great high-intensity technique for producing serious results in size and strength; your body won't become bigger and stronger if you don't push it to its limits. At the same time, going overboard (taking *every* set to failure) is counterproductive because it leads to overtraining. That's why we recommend taking no more than 1–2 sets of each exercise to failure to find the happy medium between sufficiently overloading the muscles and not breaking down the muscle fibers to the point where adequate recovery in a reasonable period (a few days) becomes virtually impossible.

3 INTENSITY PAST FAILURE

Just as training to failure is more intense than stopping short of that point, training past the point of muscle failure is more intense than simply terminating the set upon reaching

1-2
>> The max number of sets per exercise that should be taken to failure

but using them too often leads to overtraining, which can result in injury, a compromised immune system and diminished results in the gym. For beginning trainees, as well as anyone coming back from an extended hiatus from the gym, taking sets past failure isn't recommended, at least not during the first several months of training. The muscles and nervous system have enough work to do adapting to straight sets; using intensity techniques such as drop sets, rest-pauses and forced reps can be overkill and is often unnecessary for getting bigger and stronger. An important thing you'll learn as you become more experienced is when to add intensity to your training and when to back off.

The measure of intensity for a given set is whether it's taken to failure — or even past failure

failure initially. Several techniques allow you to continue doing reps after failing, including: drop sets, in which you immediately decrease the amount of weight you're lifting and continue the set without resting; rest-pauses, where you put the weight down and rest anywhere from 15–30 seconds, then do 2–3 more reps with the same weight (typically not to failure) and repeat this process 1–2 more times; and forced reps, where a partner assists you in getting anywhere from 1–3 additional reps.

In a bodybuilding workout, such techniques are the best means of maximizing training intensity. But these intensity-boosters are a double-edged sword — using them breaks down more muscle fibers and thus elicits gains in size and strength,

4 INTENSITY AT REST

Varying your rest periods between sets can greatly affect intensity. The most common way to manipulate rest in a bodybuilding-style workout is to take shorter breaks between sets (30–60 seconds as opposed to two minutes or more, as powerlifters and strength athletes often do). Decreasing rest periods prevents your muscles from recovering fully before the next set, making subsequent sets more difficult to the point that the number of reps you can do per set diminishes. For example, if you use the same weight on flat-bench dumbbell presses for three sets with only, say, 45 seconds of rest between sets, on the first set you might be able to get

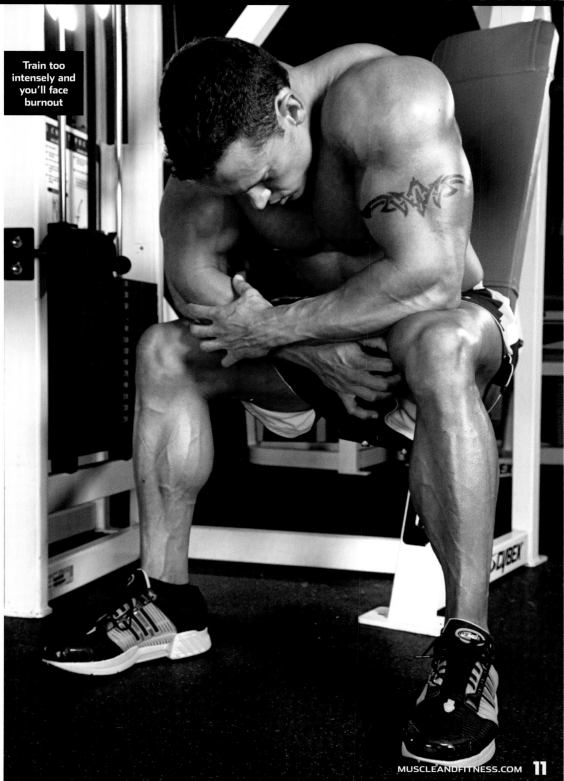

Train too intensely and you'll face burnout

12 reps, but by the third set (assuming you're training close to failure) you may get only eight reps. Since intensity was increased by minimizing rest periods, the muscles fatigued that much quicker.

There's another way to look at rest periods. Using the previous example, let's say you rested as long as two minutes between each set, which allowed you to get 12 reps on all three sets using the same weight instead of getting only eight reps on the last set. Some would say that the longer rest periods decreased intensity, yet more work was performed (more total reps were achieved with the same amount of weight), albeit over a longer period. Completing more repetitions means you stimulated the muscles that much more, which can lead to greater increases in muscle mass.

So which side of the debate is correct? Well, it intense and one of diminishing returns, the workout must be considered as a whole. In No. 2, we recommended you do no more than 1–2 sets to failure per exercise. This helps to minimize the risk of overtraining and allows you to maintain a high intensity level from beginning to end of a single workout. In addressing the latter, the more sets you take to failure early in your workout, the less intense your workout will be toward the end, as the amount of weight you can use and/or the number of reps you can perform decreases due to muscular fatigue.

Similar logic applies to overall training volume (total number of sets in a given workout). Doing too many sets in your routine drains your intensity as time lapses because of increased muscular fatigue. For example, let's compare two chest

For intensity levels to remain high, overall volume per workout needs to be kept in check

largely depends on your goals. Longer rest periods (2–3 minutes) are better for increasing strength, while resting one minute or less, even if it means using less weight or doing fewer total reps, has shown to be effective for hypertrophy (muscle growth). Since both are important, we recommend mixing both durations of rest into your program to promote varying stimuli and continued gains over the long term.

INTENSITY OF A WORKOUT
To this point, intensity has more or less been discussed on a set-by-set basis. To effectively toe the line between a training session that's sufficiently workouts, one consisting of 10 sets and the other of 20 sets. Since your muscles will be less fatigued from less work in the first workout, your last few sets will be more intense than the last few sets of the 20-set workout. This begs the question: Is it worth doing more volume in a workout if by the end of it your training intensity is largely diminished? Our contention is no, for two reasons: 1) continuing to train when stabilizer muscles are significantly fatigued can lead to injury, and 2) enhancing muscle size is dependent upon intensity, and when intensity levels are low, growth potential is equally hampered.

Bottom line, for intensity levels to remain high, overall volume per workout needs to be kept in check. After graduating from beginner status,

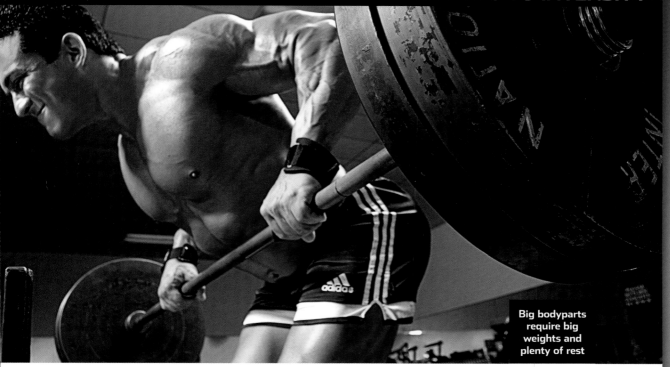

Big bodyparts require big weights and plenty of rest

each major muscle group should be trained with no more than 15 sets per workout. More than that lowers intensity, and leads to overtraining and diminished results.

6 INTENSITY OF A PROGRAM

Time to pull back and look at the bigger picture: the structure of your training program over the course of weeks, months and years, and how it affects intensity. Just as doing too many sets (especially sets to failure) in a workout decreases intensity by the end of that session, so, too, does continuously excessive volume in workout after workout negatively affect the intensity with which you're able to train day after day. Long-term overtraining zaps your energy, making every workout less effective until the body is provided ample recovery to train at maximum strength and intensity.

Ensuring this is a matter of not only keeping volume in check in every workout but also resting each bodypart sufficiently between workouts. Depending on how many sets you perform, a good rule of thumb is to rest at least two days to up to a week between training the same bodypart. If a bodypart is trained with low volume (less than five sets or so), two days of rest is probably sufficient; if you do 10–12 sets per bodypart, it probably requires 3–4 days of rest; and any more than 12 sets for one bodypart likely requires at least five days of rest. Of course, different bodyparts can be trained while others are resting, which is why you train different muscle groups on different days.

Yet just as intensity isn't always a tangible variable, we can't generalize how much volume is too much or too little for every single person. Some trainees can get away with resting only 3–4 days following an intense high-volume workout, while others may need a full week to recover. Knowing how much intensity is enough — and how much is too much — for your body is something you'll have to determine over time through trial and error.

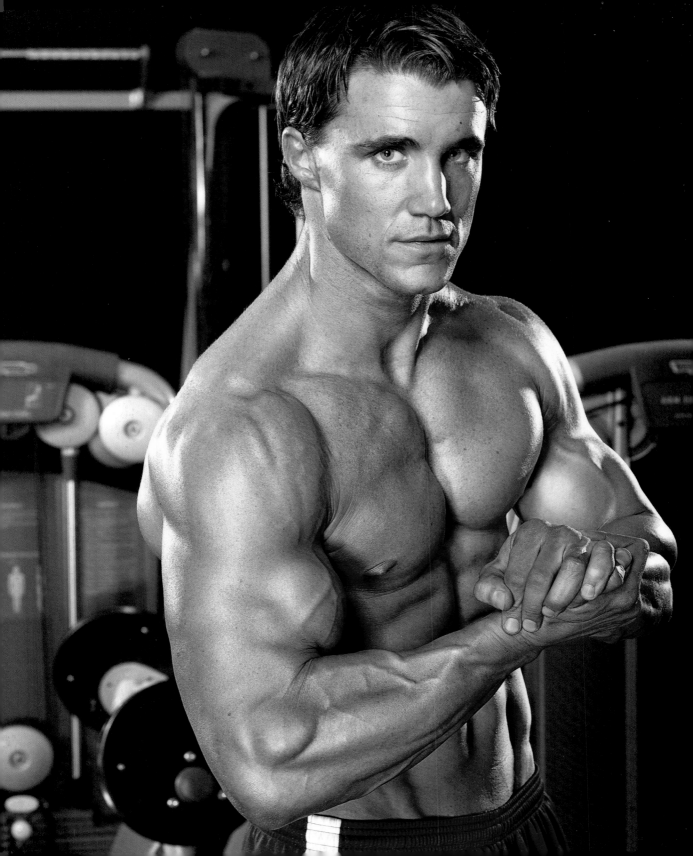

CHAPTER 2

GET LEAN WITH SUPER SETS

THIS FOUR-WEEK PROGRAM COMPOSED ENTIRELY OF SUPERSETS WILL GET YOU TIGHTER ALL OVER — AND TURN YOUR LOVE HANDLES INTO A WASHBOARD MIDSECTION

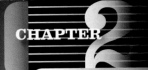

First things first. Start with the goal: burning fat, getting superlean, having a great six-pack — it's all the same. Next, determine the quickest, most effective means of achieving that goal: a fat-burning diet, yes. Sufficient cardio, definitely. And the lifting? That's easy: supersets.

Adding muscle mass by hitting the weights raises your metabolism, helping you to burn more fat in the gym and at rest. Research shows that resistance training boosts your resting metabolic rate higher and for longer than even cardio activity does. In fact, one study found that test subjects on a low-calorie diet who lifted weights experienced an actual hike in their resting metabolic rate, while the resting metabolic rate of those who did just cardio fell.

Supersets — in which you perform two exercises back to back without rest — ups the fat-burnng ante. The technique forces you to do more work in less time because you move from one exercise to the next without rest. And since each working set requires all-out effort, your calorie expenditure skyrockets!

Research concurs: The less time you spend resting between sets, the more calories you burn. Supersets are a great way to amp up your intensity, giving you a blistering workout, boosting your metabolic rate and helping you to incinerate fat faster, all in less time. That's why this training protocol is the basis of the following four-week fat-burning program. Mind you, we didn't just sprinkle in a superset here and there so you'd burn a few extra calories every workout. Each week gets progressively tougher and more effective at melting away bodyfat; in fact, Week 4 might just be the most intense four days you've ever encountered in the weight room. We like to think of this program as your love handles' worst enemy.

Supersets come in varying degrees of volume and intensity, which is clearly displayed over the four weeks of this program. Each week consists of a four-day split (Monday, Wednesday, Friday and Sunday are good choices for workout days) and will introduce a new method of supersetting, with Week 1 presenting the least challenging training sessions — not to say they're easy — and Week 4 the most demanding. Check out the rules listed below and then get started!

Supersetting Rules

» Within supersets, rest between exercises only as long as it takes you to move from one to the next. The whole point of supersetting, after all, is to ratchet up the intensity so you burn more calories and torch bodyfat. During Week 4, however, feel free to rest up to 15 seconds within the extended sets due to the extreme volume involved.

» Between supersets, rest up to two minutes during Weeks 1–3 and rest 2–3 minutes in Week 4. If you start your next superset too soon, you won't maximize your gains. Increasing intensity is one thing, but having no strength left halfway through your workout is another, so make good use of the rest intervals.

» Before every workout, thoroughly warm up each bodypart you're training that day. If it's shoulder day, do a few sets to work all three deltoid heads (middle, front and rear). A set or two of lateral raises isn't sufficient for the amount of intensity you're about to experience.

» Take each set within supersets, tri-sets and extended sets to failure. If a set calls for 10 reps, don't select a weight with which you can per-form twice that number of reps. However, use common sense: Supersetting often means you won't be able to lift as much weight as usual. Don't be afraid to decrease the resistance to reach the target number of reps.

» When supersetting opposing muscle groups (not just in this program, but anytime), don't always begin with the same bodypart. If you often superset your chest and back, for example, alternate which muscle group you train first every other workout to promote overall muscular balance in your physique.

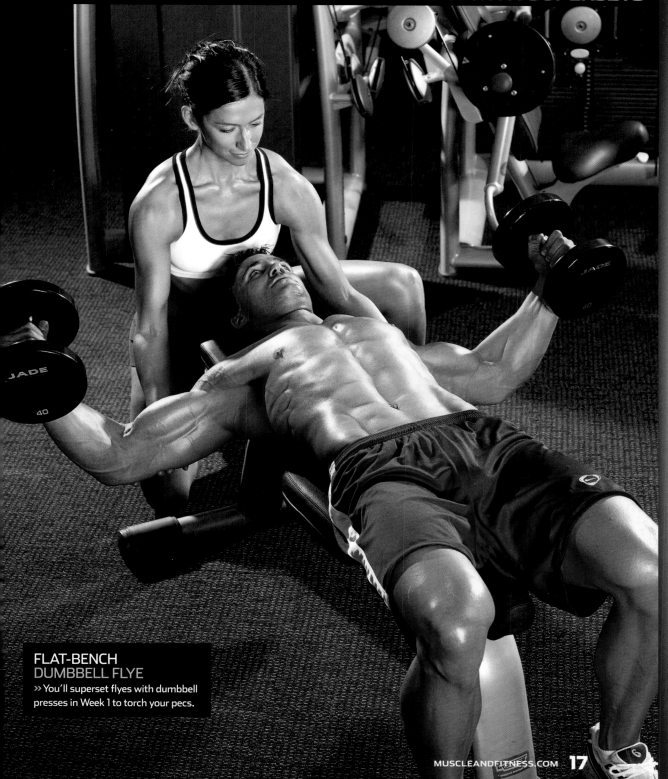

FLAT-BENCH
DUMBBELL FLYE
» You'll superset flyes with dumbbell presses in Week 1 to torch your pecs.

WEEK ONE
SAME-BODYPART SUPERSETS

>> **YOUR BASIC SUPERSET** entails performing two exercises back to back with virtually no rest in between; this combination includes two sets but counts as only one superset. (You *do* rest between each superset.) Within a superset, you'll train either the same bodypart with two exercises or perform one movement each for two different muscle groups. Week 1 employs the former, so you thoroughly exhaust each major bodypart before moving on to the next one. Almost always, the first exercise of a superset is a mass-building/compound move and the second is a single-joint isolation move; this is our way of easing you into the program.

From the start (especially if you're not accustomed to doing supersets or training with short rest periods and high reps), you'll notice an increased level of intensity in each routine compared to straight-set training. Greater intensity in the gym boosts postworkout growth-hormone levels, thus increasing muscle growth and stoking the fat-burning process.

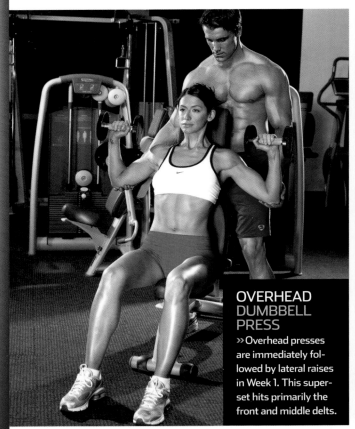

OVERHEAD DUMBBELL PRESS
>> Overhead presses are immediately followed by lateral raises in Week 1. This superset hits primarily the front and middle delts.

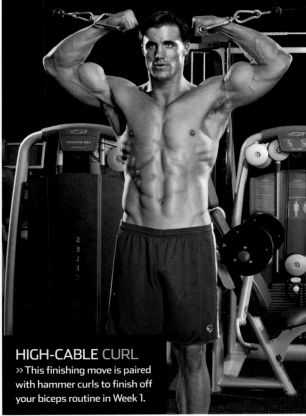

HIGH-CABLE CURL
>> This finishing move is paired with hammer curls to finish off your biceps routine in Week 1.

DAY 1

EXERCISE	SETS	REPS
CHEST		
Incline Bench Press	2	8
— superset with —		
Incline Dumbbell Flye	2	8
Flat-Bench Dumbbell Press	3	10
— superset with —		
Flat-Bench Dumbbell Flye	3	10
TRICEPS		
Bench Dip	2	8
— superset with —		
Lying Triceps Extension	2	8
Close-Grip Bench Press	2	10
— superset with —		
Pushdown	2	10

DAY 2

EXERCISE	SETS	REPS
QUADS		
Barbell Squat	3	8
— superset with —		
Leg Press	3	8
HAMSTRINGS		
Romanian Deadlift	2	12
— superset with —		
Lying Leg Curl	2	12
CALVES		
Standing Calf Raise	3	20
— superset with —		
Seated Calf Raise	3	20

DAY 3

EXERCISE	SETS	REPS
SHOULDERS		
Overhead Dumbbell Press	2	8
— superset with —		
Dumbbell Lateral Raise	2	8
Upright Row	2	10
— superset with —		
Bent-Over Lateral Raise	2	12
ABS		
Reverse Crunch	3	12
— superset with —		
Crunch	3	12
TRAPS		
Barbell Shrug	3	8
— superset with —		
Incline Dumbbell Shrug	3	8

DAY 4

EXERCISE	SETS	REPS
BACK		
Barbell Bent-Over Row	3	10
— superset with —		
Seated Row	3	10
T-Bar Row	2	12
— superset with —		
Lat Pulldown	2	12
BICEPS		
Barbell Curl	2	8
— superset with —		
Incline Dumbbell Curl	2	8
High-Cable Curl	2	10
— superset with —		
Hammer Curl	2	10

WEEK TWO

OPPOSING BODYPART SUPERSETS

>> **THESE FOUR ROUTINES** pair opposing muscle groups (for example, chest and back), except calves, which you'll train similar to Week 1. Not only does pairing save you time in the gym, but you should also be stronger on the second exercise of each superset — research shows that a muscle contracts more strongly when preceded by a contraction of its opposing (antagonist) muscle group. This added benefit could result in strength gains on top of your fat-burning ambitions.

Back shows up twice this week because shoulders don't have an obvious opposing muscle group. On Day 1, the chest and back superset movements more or less mirror each other, such as the bent-over row paired with the bench press, or the incline bench press with the seated cable row. On Day 4, your shoulder and back moves do the same, pairing exercises such as the overhead press and the lat pulldown, or the Arnold press and the chin.

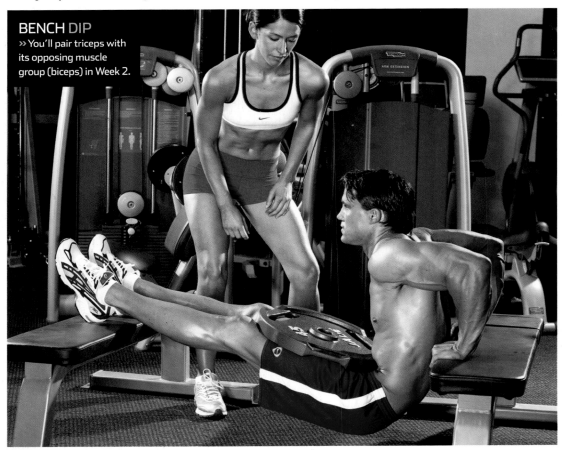

BENCH DIP
>> You'll pair triceps with its opposing muscle group (biceps) in Week 2.

DAY 1

EXERCISE	SETS	REPS
CHEST/BACK		
Barbell Bench Press	4	6
— superset with —		
Barbell Bent-Over Row	4	6
Incline Bench Press	3	8
— superset with —		
Seated Cable Row	3	8

DAY 2

EXERCISE	SETS	REPS
QUADS/HAMSTRINGS		
Smith Machine Squat	3	6
— superset with —		
Romanian Deadlift	3	6
Leg Extension	3	10
— superset with —		
Leg Curl	3	10
CALVES		
Standing Calf Raise	3	20
— superset with —		
Seated Calf Raise	3	20

DAY 3

EXERCISE	SETS	REPS
BICEPS/TRICEPS		
Preacher Curl	3	6
— superset with —		
Overhead Dumbbell Extension	3	6
Hammer Curl	3	10
— superset with —		
Bench Dip	3	10
ABS		
Cable Crunch	2	12
— superset with —		
Reverse Crunch	2	12

DAY 4

EXERCISE	SETS	REPS
SHOULDERS/BACK		
Overhead Barbell Press	3	6
— superset with —		
Lat Pulldown	3	6
Arnold Press	2	8
— superset with —		
Chin	2	8
Dumbbell Front Raise	2	10
— superset with —		
Straight-Arm Lat Pulldown	2	10

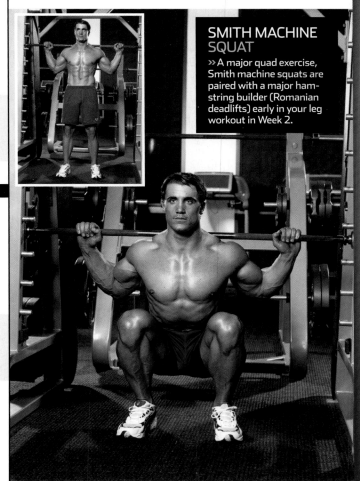

SMITH MACHINE SQUAT

>> A major quad exercise, Smith machine squats are paired with a major hamstring builder (Romanian deadlifts) early in your leg workout in Week 2.

WEEK THREE
TRI-SETS

›› **NO LONGER ARE YOUR** supersets limited to two exercises performed back to back; this week, do three exercises in a row without rest, which is known as a tri-set. Similar to Week 1, each tri-set focuses on a single bodypart; the addition of a third exercise further increases intensity and calorie burn. To avoid overtraining, perform only 2–3 tri-sets per trio of moves, whereas Weeks 1 and 2 often called for four supersets for a given pair of exercises. Utilize a broad spectrum of reps this week, sometimes going heavy and doing only four reps, and other times using less weight and reps as high as 20. This variation hits upon strength, hypertrophy and endurance in each tri-set.

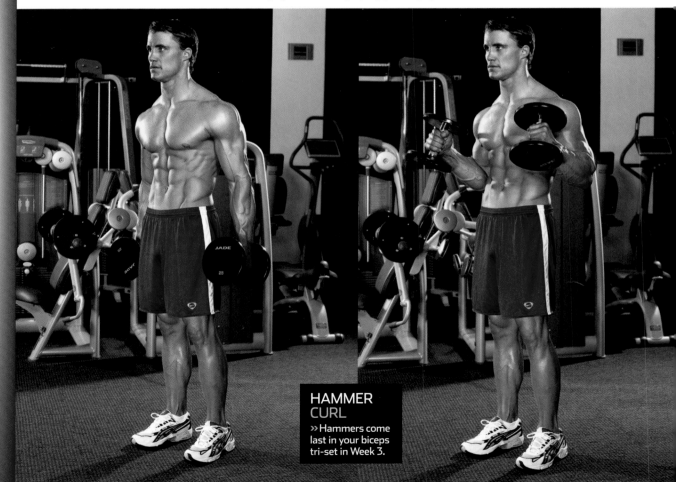

HAMMER CURL
›› Hammers come last in your biceps tri-set in Week 3.

DAY 1

EXERCISE	SETS	REPS
CHEST		
Incline Barbell Press	3	4
— tri-set with —		
Incline Dumbbell Flye	3	12
— tri-set with —		
Flat-Bench Dumbbell Flye	3	20
TRICEPS		
Lying Triceps Extension	2	4
— tri-set with —		
Pushdown	2	12
— tri-set with —		
Overhead Dumbbell Extension	2	20

DAY 2

EXERCISE	SETS	REPS
LEGS		
Barbell Squat	3	4
— tri-set with —		
Leg Press	3	12
— tri-set with —		
Leg Extension	3	20
CALVES		
Standing Calf Raise	2	12
— tri-set with —		
Seated Calf Raise	2	12
— tri-set with —		
Donkey Calf Raise	2	12

DAY 3

EXERCISE	SETS	REPS
SHOULDERS		
Seated Overhead Press	3	4
— tri-set with —		
Dumbbell Lateral Raise	3	12
— tri-set with —		
Reverse Pec-Deck Flye	3	20
TRAPS		
Barbell Shrug	2	4
— tri-set with —		
Incline Dumbbell Shrug	2	12
— tri-set with —		
Behind-the-Back Smith Machine Shrug	2	20
ABS		
Russian Twist	2	10
— tri-set with —		
Hanging Leg Raise	2	10
— tri-set with —		
Crunch	2	10

DAY 4

EXERCISE	SETS	REPS
BACK		
Chin	3	4
— tri-set with —		
Seated Row	3	12
— tri-set with —		
Straight-Arm Lat Pulldown	3	20
BICEPS		
Preacher Curl	2	4
— tri-set with —		
Standing Barbell Curl	2	12
— tri-set with —		
Hammer Curl	2	20

DUMBBELL LATERAL RAISE
» Fry your delts as part of your next shoulder tri-set.

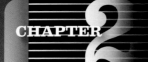
WEEK FOUR

EXTENDED SETS

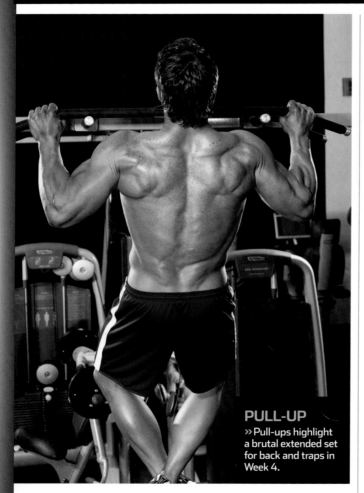

PULL-UP
» Pull-ups highlight a brutal extended set for back and traps in Week 4.

» **WE WON'T SUGARCOAT IT:** This week is downright brutal. It calls into play extended sets, which for our program comprise up to eight different exercises you perform consecutively. However, an extended set differs from a superset or tri-set in that many of the exercises used — though similar — involve a change of angle or grip. Take, for

example, the first extended set of chest moves on Day 1: The first three exercises include the incline dumbbell press, flat-bench dumbbell press and decline dumbbell press. Although these are technically different exercises, the motion — pressing the weights over your chest with your pec muscles — remains virtually the same. After these exercises, you move on to the next two, both of which involve working the chest with cable movements. As you complete the sequence of exercises in your extended sets, the minimal changes required act to increase the intensity as you blast a wide variety of muscle fibers in rapid succession.

The order in which you perform the movements in extended sets is crucial. In the aforementioned example, notice how the toughest variation of the three pressing movements (incline) is done first, while the easiest (decline) comes last. Getting the most out of extended sets relies on increasing your body's mechanical advantage from set to set. Imagine if you did these exercises in the reverse order, from easiest to hardest. Sure, you could perform more reps on the decline bench, but by the time you got to the incline, you'd be so fatigued that getting an appreciable number of reps on the hardest of the three moves would be unthinkable.

For each exercise in an extended set, select a weight that's approximately your five-rep max (except for calves), and take each set within the extended set to failure.

There you have it! Four weeks of supersets that'll help you get superlean. Remember, for you to find success with this program, you must follow the instructions carefully and adhere to the appropriate rest protocols within and between each superset. So what are you waiting for? Get started toward super results!

DAY 1

EXERCISE	SETS	REPS
CHEST		
Incline Dumbbell Press	2	5
— followed by —		
Flat-Bench Dumbbell Press	2	5
— followed by —		
Decline Dumbbell Press	2	5
— followed by —		
Low-Cable Crossover	2	5
— followed by —		
High-Cable Crossover	2	5
TRICEPS/BICEPS		
Dumbbell Overhead Extension	2	5
— followed by —		
Pushdown	2	5
— followed by —		
Reverse-Grip Curl	2	5
— followed by —		
Barbell Curl	2	5
— followed by —		
Hammer Curl	2	5

DAY 2

EXERCISE	SETS	REPS
QUADS/HAMSTRINGS		
Front Squat	3	5
— followed by —		
Smith Machine Squat	3	5
— followed by —		
Romanian Deadlift	3	5
— followed by —		
Lying Leg Curl	3	5
CALVES		
Standing Calf Raise	3	20
— superset with —		
Seated Calf Raise	3	20

DAY 3

EXERCISE	SETS	REPS
SHOULDERS		
Dumbbell Front Raise	2	5
— followed by —		
Upright Row	2	5
— followed by —		
Barbell Overhead Press	2	5
— followed by —		
Bent-Over Lateral Raise	2	5
— followed by —		
Dumbbell Lateral Raise	2	5
ABS		
Reverse Crunch	3	12
— superset with —		
Crunch	3	12

DAY 4

EXERCISE	SETS	REPS
BACK/TRAPS		
Barbell Row	2	5
— followed by —		
Reverse-Grip Barbell Row	2	5
— followed by —		
Smith Machine Behind-the-Back Shrug	2	5
— followed by —		
Barbell Shrug	2	5
Pull-Up	2	5
— followed by —		
Chin	2	5
— followed by —		
Incline Dumbbell Shrug	2	5

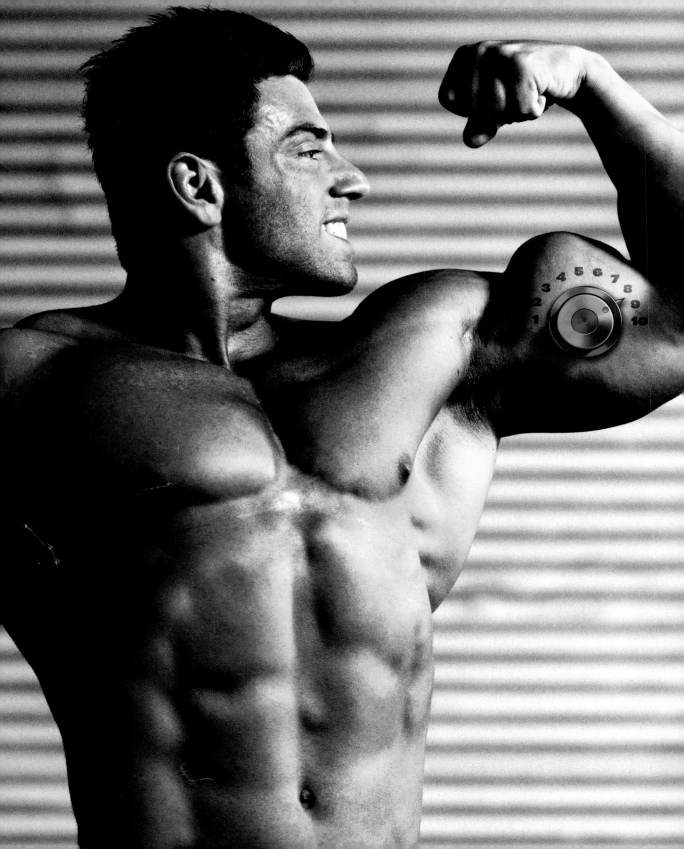

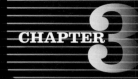

PUMPED
VOLUME

THIS BARE-BONES, SINGLE-EXERCISE APPROACH WILL HELP VOLUMIZE YOUR WORKOUT AND YOUR PHYSIQUE

Over time, you've come to love the cathartic release of hitting the iron, your day's troubles fading away with each rep. Tonight, you have a full assortment of presses and flyes in store for your chest to hit your pecs from every conceivable angle. Who cares if your workday sucked? You'll spend tonight growing, and (thankfully) tomorrow's a fresh start.

With optimism in tow, you head to the gym. But once you get there, your gloom is renewed: Two guys are waiting at the incline bench, the Hammer Strength machines are all being used, a trainer is doing more chatting than training with a woman at the pec deck, and the dumbbells you were hoping to get at are being monopolized by some local high school football players. The gym's lone Smith machine bears a "Do Not Use" sign while a technician re-tracks the barbell.

Still, there's no need to go out of your skull and start choking people with your towel. You may not be able to bounce around the gym in quite the way you intended, but here's the good news: You don't need to. Choosing one major exercise for a bodypart and then training it to exhaustion with that one move not only saves you the headaches of gym traffic but can actually help you recruit, exhaust and develop more total muscle fibers. Plus, this "one and done" approach means

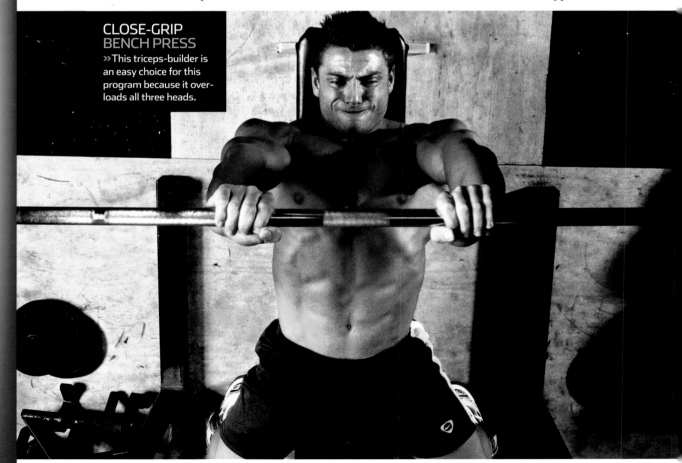

CLOSE-GRIP BENCH PRESS
»This triceps-builder is an easy choice for this program because it overloads all three heads.

you can work each muscle group twice per week — simply choose another emphasis your next time through. This system of training saves time and acts as a type of shock routine, but like all shock routines, it should be followed for only a specific time period; in this case, we recommend four weeks.

Thus, our four-week "Pumped Volume" workout focuses on multiple sets of one movement for each bodypart per trip to the gym. Three or four sets of an exercise can be effective, but a higher concentration of work (for this program the range is 8–15 sets) through a particular range of motion will leave little doubt that you've completely taxed every single fiber in the targeted muscle. Someone looking to add mass to his upper chest might frontload his workout with a few extra sets of inclines before moving on to flat-bench, decline or flye moves. Think about how much more growth that lifter could coax out of those upper-chest fibers with a full 12 hard sets of one incline exercise!

So don't fret, oh mighty hater of crowds. By pumping up the volume of sets you spend on one exercise, you'll be able to pump up your physique like never before, without having to wipe and walk every 10 minutes and without having to wait on equipment. Your training is already on blast — now it's time to turn things up a bit.

DAILY (LACK OF) VARIETY

Doing various exercises for a particular bodypart is great because you get to tax the muscle from different angles and in different ways. Varying stimuli challenge your muscles and your nervous system to adapt, learn and respond. But sometimes doing a lift-a-palooza for your back, for example, may be less effective than picking one exercise and doing it for more sets.

Consider that a typical, well-balanced back day usually includes some kind of heavy row for back thickness, a variation of a pulldown for width and perhaps a finisher such as back extensions or straight-arm pulldowns for definition. In this scenario, however, the various areas of your back get only a few sets each of intense, targeted work.

Picking one movement for your back — such as the lat pulldown — and simply taking it to the limit with eight or more sets will eliminate the speculation on muscle recruitment. Do that many sets with one move and you'll know that you've punished each muscle fiber beyond anything it's accustomed to.

Some bodybuilders also favor this approach for determining an exercise's worth to their program. Execute that many sets of one movement and, within 24–48 hours, muscle soreness will tell you what nooks and crannies it hits.

Resistance training helps signal the release of growth hormone (GH), a key factor in muscle growth, strength gains and fat-burning. If your typical weight workout produces a wave of GH, the "Pumped Volume" approach is a tsunami. As the reps and sets increase over the four-week period, your body will be forced to release greater amounts of this precious hormone because performing more reps increases the amount of lactic acid your muscles produce, and high levels of

The Pumped Volume Program

» In this four-week full-body blast designed to exhaust more total fibers of the targeted muscle group, you'll train each muscle group twice per week, alternating between two different exercises per bodypart. Use the following three-day split — done twice per week — for a total of six training days per week.

TRAINING SPLIT

DAY	BODYPARTS TRAINED
1	Chest, biceps
2	Shoulders, legs, calves
3	Back, triceps, abs
4	Chest, biceps
5	Shoulders, legs, calves
6	Back, triceps, abs
7	Rest

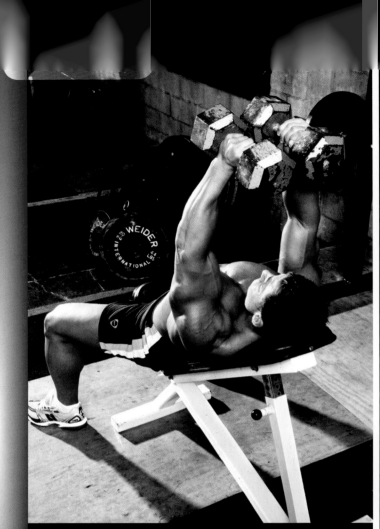

INCLINE FLYE
›› Done with proper resistance, the incline flye can be much more than a finishing movement — it can help thicken your upper pecs.

HANGING LEG RAISE
›› Your crunch marathons will be replaced by more challenging moves like this one and the cable crunch.

lactic acid stimulate the release of GH. All you have to do is sit back and enjoy the results (and perhaps keep your massage therapist's number on speed dial).

An additional benefit is that the repeated performance of the same exercise set after set will help you program your nervous system to better synchronize the contraction of each muscle fiber needed during that exercise. Better synchronization means a better working system, and that means greater strength gains for you over the course of this four-week program.

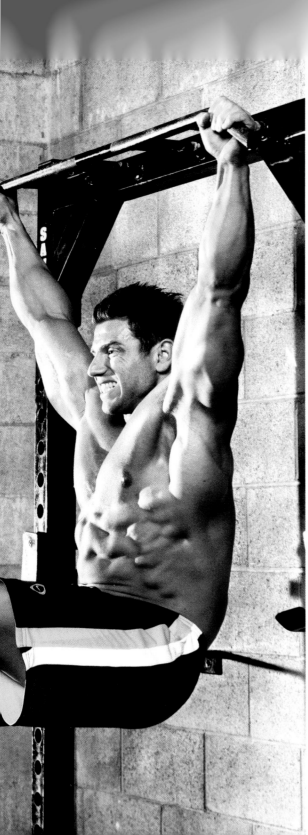

WEEK ONE

MONDAY

MUSCLE GROUP	EXERCISE	SETS/REPS	REST
CHEST	Bench Press	8/8	2 min.
BICEPS	Preacher Curl	8/8	2 min.

TUESDAY

MUSCLE GROUP	EXERCISE	SETS/REPS	REST
SHOULDERS	Lateral Raise	8/8	2 min.
LEGS	Squat	8/8	2 min.
CALVES	Standing Calf Raise	8/8	1 min.

WEDNESDAY

MUSCLE GROUP	EXERCISE	SETS/REPS	REST
BACK	Bent-Over Row	8/8	2 min.
TRICEPS	Pushdown	8/8	2 min.
ABS	Hanging Leg Raise	8/8	1 min.

THURSDAY

MUSCLE GROUP	EXERCISE	SETS/REPS	REST
CHEST	Incline Flye	8/8	2 min.
BICEPS	Barbell Curl	8/8	2 min.

FRIDAY

MUSCLE GROUP	EXERCISE	SETS/REPS	REST
SHOULDERS	Dumbbell Overhead Press	8/8	2 min.
LEGS	Leg Press	8/8	2 min.
CALVES	Seated Calf Raise	8/8	1 min.

SATURDAY

MUSCLE GROUP	EXERCISE	SETS/REPS	REST
BACK	Pulldown	8/8	2 min.
TRICEPS	Close-Grip Bench Press	8/8	2 min.
ABS	Cable Crunch	8/8	1 min.

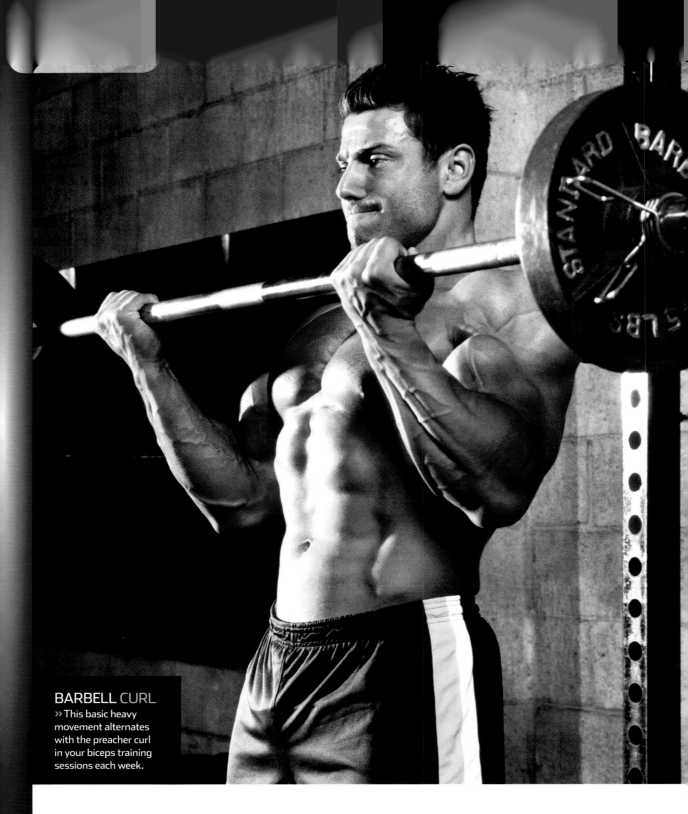

BARBELL CURL

» This basic heavy movement alternates with the preacher curl in your biceps training sessions each week.

ADJUSTING THE VOLUME

"Pumped Volume" is slightly more complicated than saying, "Go do 10 sets of 10 barbell curls," but not so much that your brain starts to hurt. Consider a few factors when diving into this program.

>> **Muscle groupings.** Because of the brutality of the program, you'll pair nonassisting muscle groups such as chest and biceps, back and triceps, shoulders and legs. This will help to ensure that you aren't fatiguing the targeted muscles ahead of a working set.

>> **Weight selection.** Since you'll use the same weight for each set, it's important to get it right. Each week, you'll choose a weight that's about 90%–95% of your prescribed rep max (RM). For example, in Week 1 when you do eight reps per set, if your 8RM on the bench press is 200 pounds, you should use 180–190 pounds on all eight sets. Make sure, however, that you stop at the set rep range. The weight may feel a bit light the first few sets, but remember that you have several sets left and, after a while, your train-past-failure bravado will be wasted on sloppy or incomplete sets.

Hitting that number is all you need to be concerned with. If possible, have a spotter on hand to help you reach your target number on the latter sets. Solo trainees can try the rest-pause method — set down the weight for 10–15 seconds and come back to it as many times as is necessary to complete the set.

>> **Be explosive early.** On your first few sets of each exercise, perform explosive but controlled reps to recruit as many fast-twitch fibers as possible. These are the strongest fibers at your disposal and have the greatest potential for growth.

>> **What to expect.** If you've never trained like this before, it's important to know what you're in for. For your first few sets, the weight may feel light or, at the very least, manageable. That should translate well into the quicker-paced reps of your first 4–5 sets. As you fatigue, your muscles

WEEK TWO

MONDAY

MUSCLE GROUP	EXERCISE	SETS/REPS	REST
CHEST	Incline Flye	10/10	2 min.
BICEPS	Barbell Curl	10/10	2 min.

TUESDAY

MUSCLE GROUP	EXERCISE	SETS/REPS	REST
SHOULDERS	Dumbbell Overhead Press	10/10	2 min.
LEGS	Leg Press	10/10	2 min.
CALVES	Seated Calf Raise	10/10	1 min.

WEDNESDAY

MUSCLE GROUP	EXERCISE	SETS/REPS	REST
BACK	Pulldown	10/10	2 min.
TRICEPS	Close-Grip Bench Press	10/10	2 min.
ABS	Cable Crunch	10/10	1 min.

THURSDAY

MUSCLE GROUP	EXERCISE	SETS/REPS	REST
CHEST	Bench Press	10/10	2 min.
BICEPS	Preacher Curl	10/10	2 min.

FRIDAY

MUSCLE GROUP	EXERCISE	SETS/REPS	REST
SHOULDERS	Lateral Raise	10/10	2 min.
LEGS	Squat	10/10	2 min.
CALVES	Standing Calf Raise	10/10	1 min.

SATURDAY

MUSCLE GROUP	EXERCISE	SETS/REPS	REST
BACK	Bent-Over Row	10/10	2 min.
TRICEPS	Pushdown	10/10	2 min.
ABS	Hanging Leg Raise	10/10	1 min.

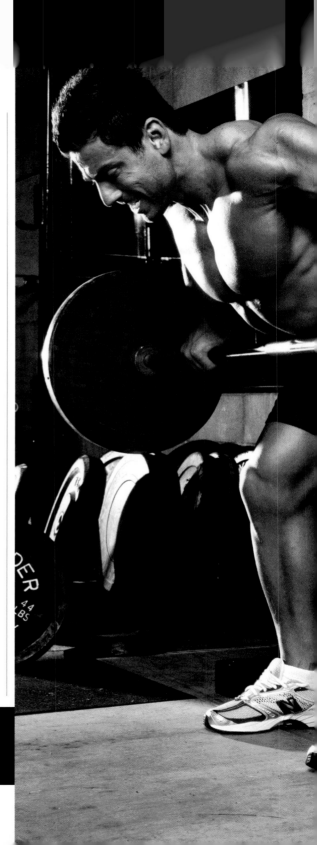

will start to bake with lactic acid buildup. The good news is that lactic acid indicates your body is signaling for an increase in GH. In these middle sets, you may find that the reps come more slowly and that rest-pause or forced reps with a spotter are necessary to reach your target number. Anecdotally, many bodybuilders report that this slow-mo subsides around the eighth set and you may once again find your groove near the finish line.

>> **Rest right.** Although the technique is intense and you can expect to lean up a bit from it, be sure to get in the proper rest between sets to maximize recuperation. In this program, that's usually 1–2 minutes. It may be tempting to decrease the rest periods and chase the pump — you'll be sporting hoselike vascularity after a few runs through this type of training — but don't give into the temptation. Rest is key. You want to get through the whole workout, right?

>> **Be angular.** Similar workouts of yesteryear would lock you into one exercise for all four weeks. But since we've doubled up your sessions per week per bodypart, our program allows you to incorporate a second exercise to promote strength through a different plane and bring more muscle into play. Using chest as an example, you'll perform barbell bench presses one day and incline flyes on another. The increased volume through these varied yet basic movements will allow you to hit more total fibers — and thus grow more muscle — than you might in a traditional single-exercise program.

PUMP TO PERFECTION

On the surface, this program might seem pretty unsophisticated. The results it yields, however,

BENT-OVER ROW
>> This back-training staple helps you build depth and density. Combine these with width-building pulldowns for complete growth.

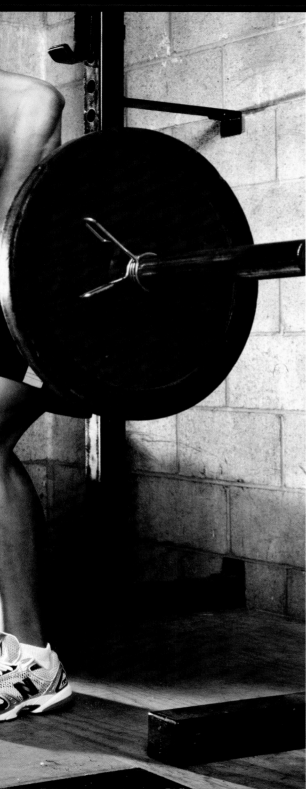

WEEK THREE

MONDAY

MUSCLE GROUP	EXERCISE	SETS/REPS	REST
CHEST	Bench Press	12/12	2 min.
BICEPS	Preacher Curl	12/12	2 min.

TUESDAY

MUSCLE GROUP	EXERCISE	SETS/REPS	REST
SHOULDERS	Lateral Raise	12/12	2 min.
LEGS	Squat	12/12	2 min.
CALVES	Standing Calf Raise	12/12	1 min.

WEDNESDAY

MUSCLE GROUP	EXERCISE	SETS/REPS	REST
BACK	Bent-Over Row	12/12	2 min.
TRICEPS	Pushdown	12/12	2 min.
ABS	Hanging Leg Raise	12/12	1 min.

THURSDAY

MUSCLE GROUP	EXERCISE	SETS/REPS	REST
CHEST	Incline Flye	12/12	2 min.
BICEPS	Barbell Curl	12/12	2 min.

FRIDAY

MUSCLE GROUP	EXERCISE	SETS/REPS	REST
SHOULDERS	Dumbbell Overhead Press	12/12	2 min.
LEGS	Leg Press	12/12	2 min.
CALVES	Seated Calf Raise	12/12	1 min.

SATURDAY

MUSCLE GROUP	EXERCISE	SETS/REPS	REST
BACK	Pulldown	12/12	2 min.
TRICEPS	Close-Grip Bench Press	12/12	2 min.
ABS	Cable Crunch	12/12	1 min.

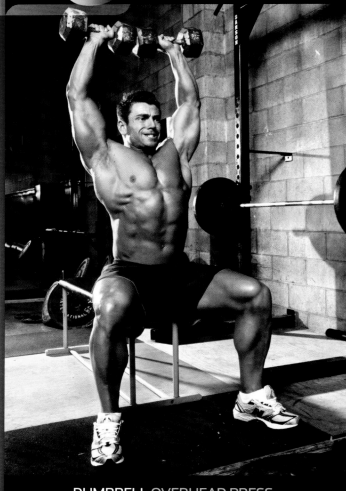

CHAPTER 3

DUMBBELL OVERHEAD PRESS
» Your front delts will be issued a beating with 8–15 sets of this move. The focus shifts to your middle delts in the next shoulder session.

are anything but. The main benefit of sticking to a single exercise for a muscle group is simple: You'll maximally recruit all of the muscle fibers that are used to complete that move.

But you don't have to be a one-exercise kind of guy forever. In fact, you should go back to a normal routine of 3–5 exercises per bodypart at the end of the four weeks. With the gains you reap from the "Pumped Volume" program, you're sure to be stronger, harder and leaner when you tackle your garden-variety routine.

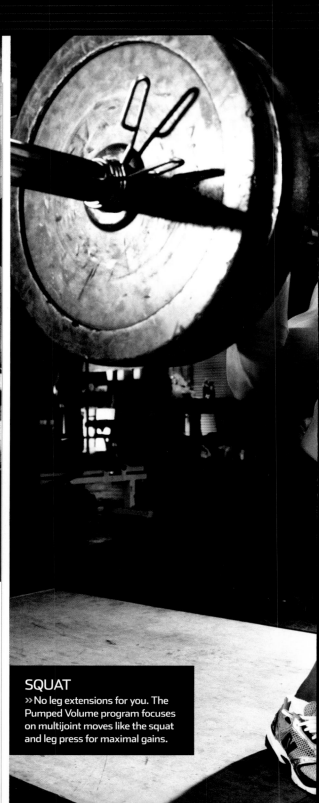

SQUAT
» No leg extensions for you. The Pumped Volume program focuses on multijoint moves like the squat and leg press for maximal gains.

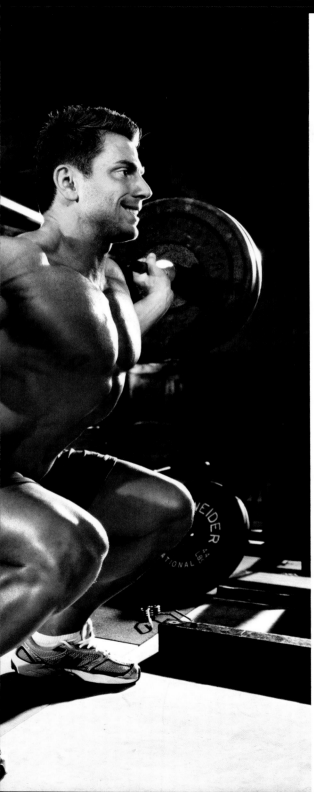

WEEK FOUR

MONDAY

MUSCLE GROUP	EXERCISE	SETS/REPS	REST
CHEST	Incline Flye	10/15	2 min.
BICEPS	Barbell Curl	10/15	2 min.

TUESDAY

MUSCLE GROUP	EXERCISE	SETS/REPS	REST
SHOULDERS	Dumbbell Overhead Press	10/15	2 min.
LEGS	Leg Press	10/15	2 min.
CALVES	Seated Calf Raise	10/15	1 min.

WEDNESDAY

MUSCLE GROUP	EXERCISE	SETS/REPS	REST
BACK	Pulldown	10/15	2 min.
TRICEPS	Close-Grip Bench Press	10/15	2 min.
ABS	Cable Crunch	10/15	1 min.

THURSDAY

MUSCLE GROUP	EXERCISE	SETS/REPS	REST
CHEST	Bench Press	10/15	2 min.
BICEPS	Preacher Curl	10/15	2 min.

FRIDAY

MUSCLE GROUP	EXERCISE	SETS/REPS	REST
SHOULDERS	Lateral Raise	10/15	2 min.
LEGS	Squat	10/15	2 min.
CALVES	Standing Calf Raise	10/15	1 min.

SATURDAY

MUSCLE GROUP	EXERCISE	SETS/REPS	REST
BACK	Bent-Over Row	10/15	2 min.
TRICEPS	Pushdown	10/15	2 min.
ABS	Hanging Leg Raise	10/15	1 min.

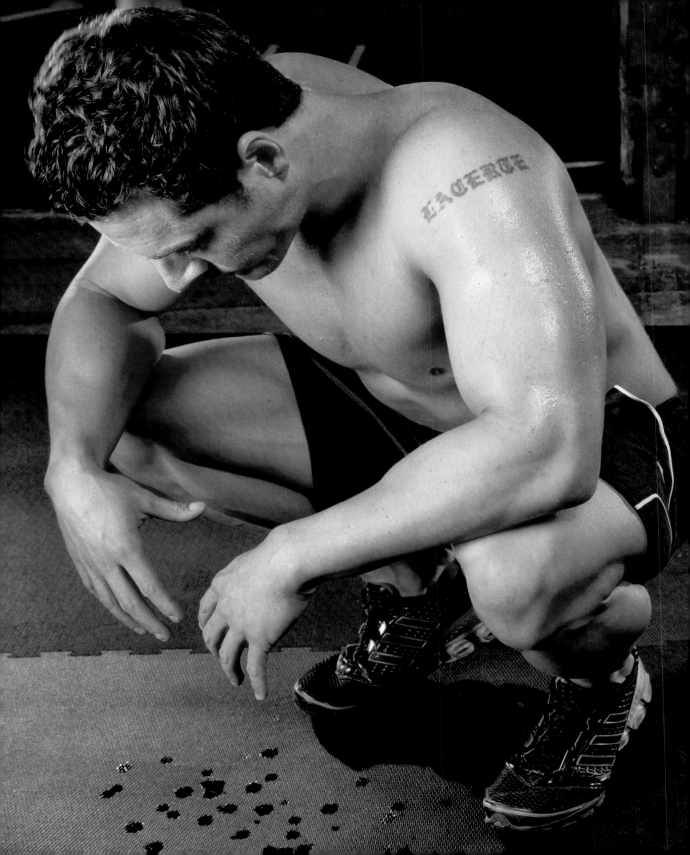

20/10
A PAIN
ODYSSEY

CREATED IN A JAPANESE SPORTS LAB, THIS HIGH-INTENSITY INTERVAL METHOD WILL BURN BODYFAT WHILE IT BUILDS MUSCLE

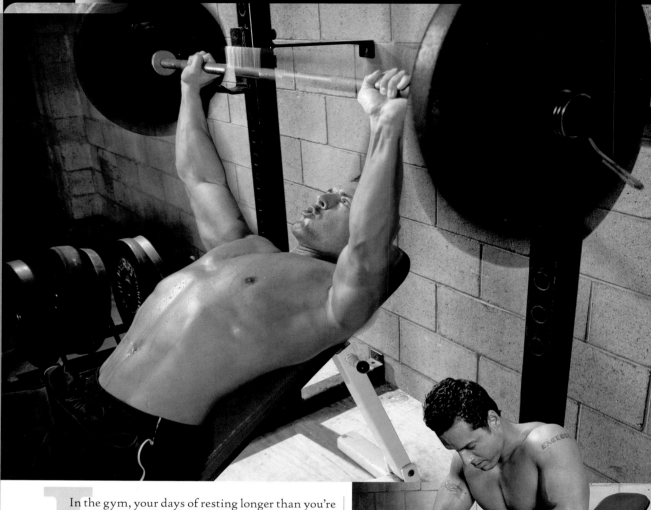

In the gym, your days of resting longer than you're actually lifting are history. Doing a set that lasts 20–30 seconds, then taking a 1–2-minute breather before another half-minute set? No more. Gone. Sayonara. Well, at least for now.

Your sets and rest periods are about to flip, and you'll be lifting for twice as long as you break. Here's what's in store: Short rest periods and high-rep sets performed at such an intensity that you'll use roughly half your normal weight. You'll burn bodyfat, your muscles will grow, you'll get an aerobic workout, and you'll increase strength and power. But it all comes at a price, and the only currency accepted is pain. It's a program as unique as its name: Tabata.

TABATA TIME

WORKOUT 1: CHEST, ABS

EXERCISE	SETS/TIME	REST[1]
CHEST		
Push-Up	8/20 sec.	10 sec.
Incline Bench Press	8/20 sec.	10 sec.
Flat-Bench Dumbbell Press	8/20 sec.	10 sec.
Cable Crossover	8/20 sec.	10 sec.
ABS		
Reverse Crunch	8/20 sec.	10 sec.
Crunch	8/20 sec.	10 sec.

WORKOUT 2: LEGS, CALVES

EXERCISE	SETS/TIME	REST[1]
QUADS/GLUTES/HAMSTRINGS		
Squat	8/20 sec.	10 sec.
Leg Press	8/20 sec.	10 sec.
Leg Extension	8/20 sec.	10 sec.
Leg Curl	8/20 sec.	10 sec.
CALVES		
Standing Calf Raise	8/20 sec.	10 sec.
Seated Calf Raise	8/20 sec.	10 sec.

WORKOUT 3: SHOULDERS, TRAPS

EXERCISE	SETS/TIME	REST[1]
SHOULDERS		
Smith Machine Overhead Press	8/20 sec.	10 sec.
Smith Machine Upright Row	8/20 sec.	10 sec.
Lateral Raise	8/20 sec.	10 sec.
Reverse Pec-Deck Flye	8/20 sec.	10 sec.
TRAPS		
Barbell Shrug	8/20 sec.	10 sec.
Dumbbell Shrug	8/20 sec.	10 sec.

WORKOUT 4: BACK, ABS

EXERCISE	SETS/TIME	REST[1]
BACK		
Bent-Over Row	8/20 sec.	10 sec.
Lat Pulldown	8/20 sec.	10 sec.
Seated Row	8/20 sec.	10 sec.
Straight-Arm Pulldown	8/20 sec.	10 sec.
ABS		
Alternating Oblique Crunch	8/20 sec.	10 sec.
Cable Crunch	8/20 sec.	10 sec.

[1] Rest 2–3 minutes between exercises.

WORKOUT 5: TRI'S, BI'S, FOREARMS

EXERCISE	SETS/TIME	REST[1]
TRICEPS		
Lying Triceps Extension	8/20 sec.	10 sec.
Pressdown	8/20 sec.	10 sec.
Overhead Cable Extension	8/20 sec.	10 sec.
BICEPS		
Barbell Curl	8/20 sec.	10 sec.
Incline Dumbbell Curl	8/20 sec.	10 sec.
Hammer Curl	8/20 sec.	10 sec.
FOREARMS		
Wrist Curl	8/20 sec.	10 sec.
Reverse Wrist Curl	8/20 sec.	10 sec.

[1] Rest 2–3 minutes between exercises.

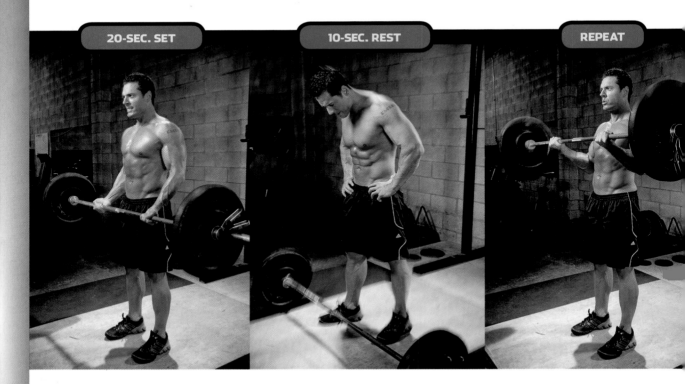

20-SEC. SET   **10-SEC. REST**   **REPEAT**

TIMING IS EVERYTHING

For the weightlifter, the measurables boil down to sets, reps and the amount of weight used. How many sets did I do? How many reps per set? And most important, how heavy did I go? But sometimes, when your results have hit a plateau, you need to think outside the box. Inside the box is this: Do a set of 8–10 reps, rest a minute, do another set of 8–10 reps, rest a minute. Repeat indefinitely. Not that anything is inherently wrong with this style of training, unless you've been doing it for years, not to mention decades.

Tabata Interval Training is so far out of the three-sets-of-10-reps box it doesn't even speak the same language. Using Tabata means alternating 20 seconds of exercise with 10 seconds of rest, non-stop, for eight sets. Unlike the high-intensity interval training we typically prescribe for cardio, but similar in its fat-burning effectiveness, this style of training can be adapted to any exercise: dumbbell presses, barbell rows, jumping rope, rowing, push-ups, you name it. And in true M&F fashion, we've designed a Tabata Interval Training program that's so effective, yet so grueling, that you'll thank us while you're hating us (or maybe a day or two later).

The results will be well worth the pain. The extremely short rest periods and seemingly constant reps are perfect for melting away bodyfat. Yet despite the light weight you'll be using — 50%–75% of what you'd use for a typical set of 8–12 reps, depending on the exercise — Tabata will take your muscle growth to new heights.

THE SCIENCE OF TABATA

Tabata Intervals were named after the Japanese scientist who first designed them: Izumi Tabata,

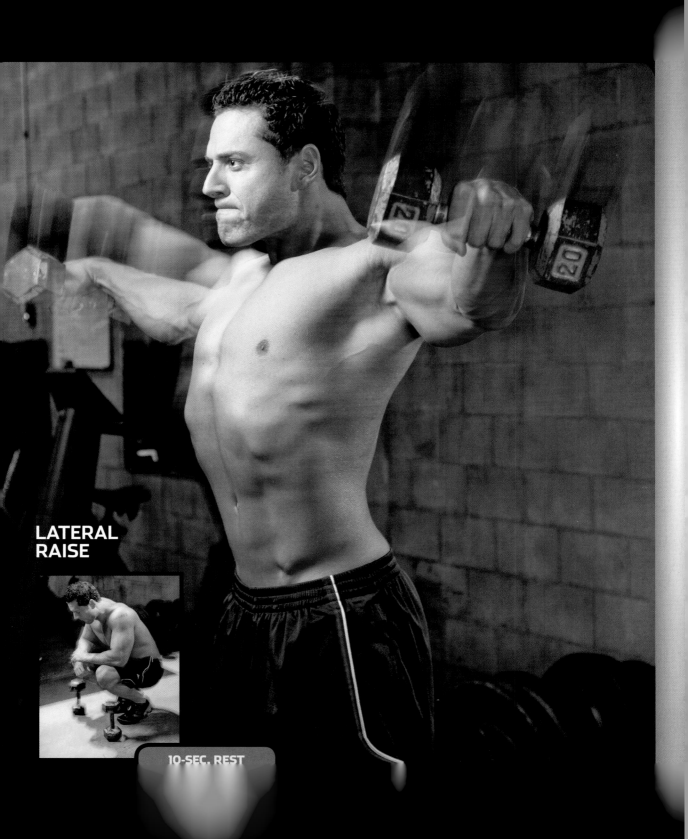

LATERAL RAISE

10-SEC. REST

PUSHDOWN

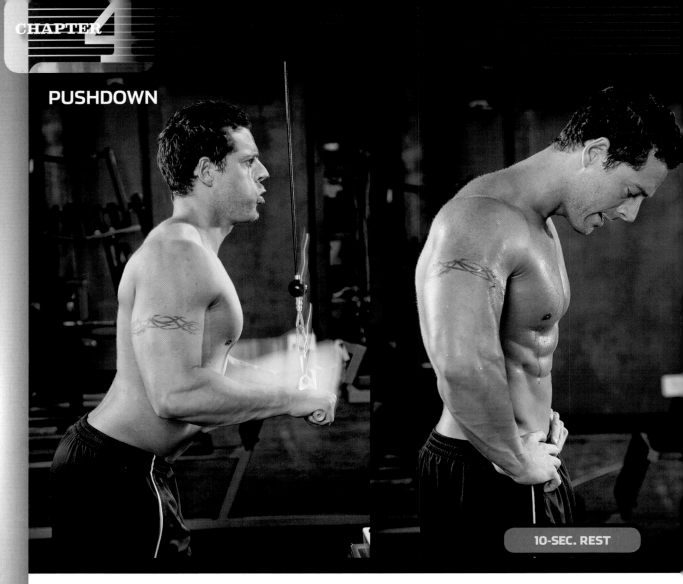

10-SEC. REST

PhD. As the story goes, Dr. T was looking for a method of gym training that would give the Japanese national speed-skating team an edge on the ice. He discovered that when his athletes performed eight cycles of 20-second high-intensity bouts followed by 10 seconds of rest, they increased both their aerobic (endurance) capacity and anaerobic (quick power) output — two things speed skaters need to be successful, but which typically don't go hand in hand. In other words, training one usually means the other is taking a back seat.

Not with Tabata. Whether you're a cyclist or a powerlifter, a boxer or a ballplayer, Tabata Interval Training offers the unique benefit of training both major metabolic pathways: those that provide endurance and those that create explosive energy.

What's in it for you? Since it enhances endurance, Tabata boosts your body's ability to burn more bodyfat. And since it bolsters explosiveness, the kind you use in a typical set of bench presses, squats or deadlifts, it can help you get more reps with a given weight and/or use more weight to perform a given number of reps. So what used to be a set of 10 reps with 200 pounds could soon be 10 reps with 225. This crosses over not only to more strength but also more growth, since a greater

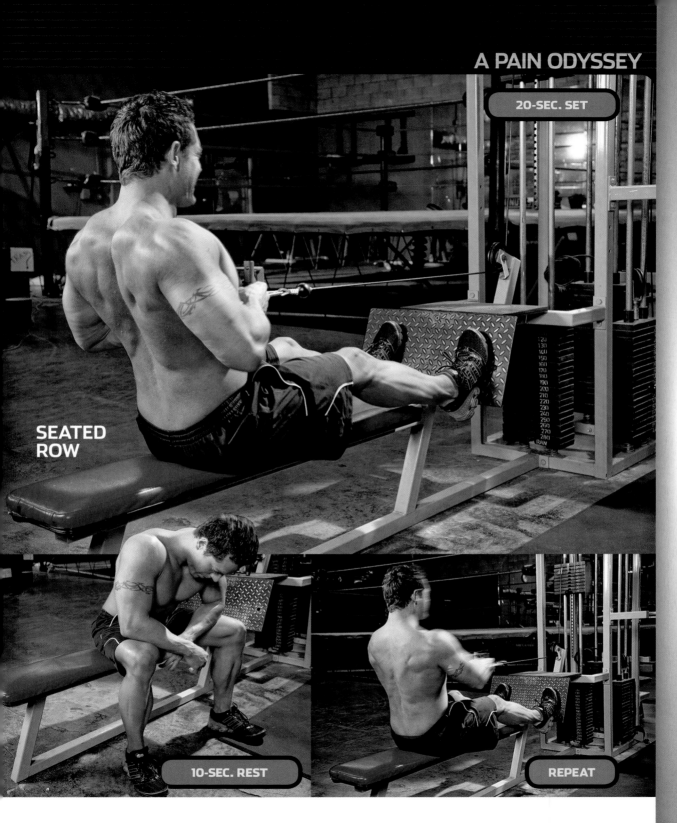

A PAIN ODYSSEY

20-SEC. SET

SEATED
ROW

10-SEC. REST

REPEAT

PUSH-UP

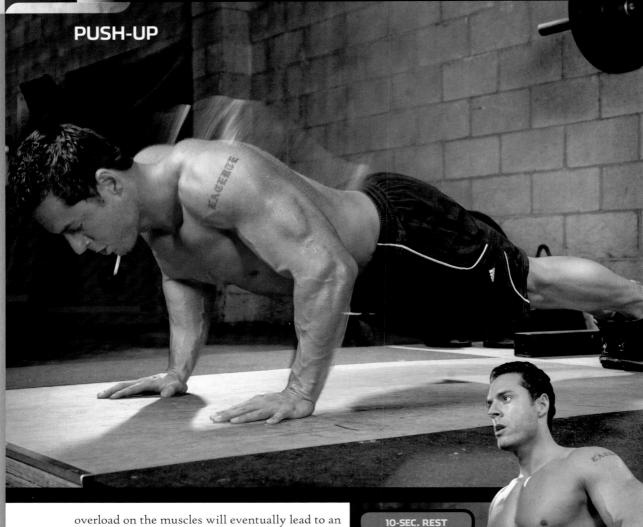

10-SEC. REST

overload on the muscles will eventually lead to an increase in their size.

The benefits don't end there. Because of a Tabata program's relatively high rep counts and extremely short rest periods, you'll actually increase the number of blood vessels feeding your muscle fibers. This will help deliver more nutrients, oxygen and anabolic hormones to the muscles, which means you'll have more energy during workouts, not to mention better recovery and growth when the session's over. And best of all, at least for those among us who loathe treadmills and elliptical machines, is the fact that Tabata counts as a cardio workout as well.

CABLE CRUNCH

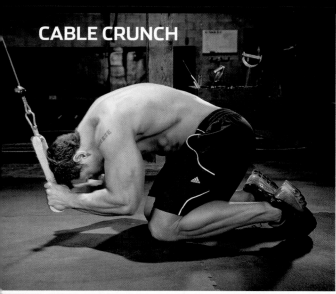

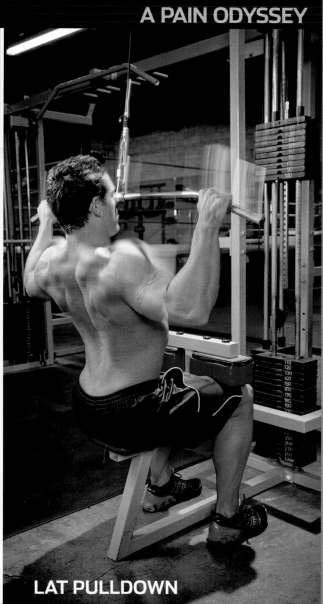

LEG CURL

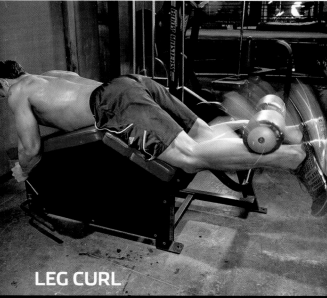

LAT PULLDOWN

TABATA, ONLY TOUGHER

Dr. T probably never envisioned his intervals being performed at such a high volume. While most Tabata practitioners focus on one exercise per major muscle group, we've revised the concept to include several exercises per bodypart. When you reach the end of each workout, you'll be wiped out like never before.

In the program that begins on page 41, you'll do 2–4 exercises Tabata-style per muscle group. Do each exercise for eight sets of 20 seconds, performing as many reps as possible (your numbers will vary, depending on individual rep speed and fatigue levels), with only 10 seconds of rest between each set. Once you complete eight sets of a given exercise, rest 2–3 minutes (if you have a training partner, you'll rest the four minutes it takes him to complete his eight sets), then repeat for the next exercise.

If you have a training partner, he can time your sets and rest periods, telling you when to start and stop. If you train solo, however, keeping time can get tricky. We suggest you use an interval timer (such as those made by Gymboss or Everlast) that allows you to set customized interval times so that the watch beeps or vibrates when your 20-second set is over and then goes off again 10 seconds later. Otherwise, find a wall clock or sneak

weight for each exercise. When you find a weight that allows you to complete a full 20 seconds of reps for the first five or six sets but has you failing on the last two or three sets, you've found the perfect resistance. Your goal, then, will be to complete the 20 seconds of reps for all eight sets (and stay true to the 10-second rest periods) before increasing the weight. While you may be able to work for each of the 20-second intervals, be prepared for your rep count to drop precipitously as you slog through the sets of each exercise.

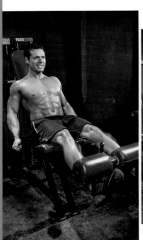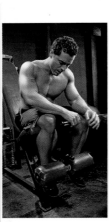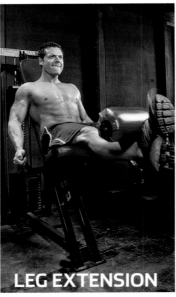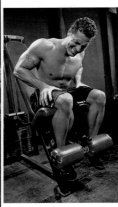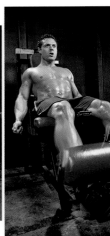

LEG EXTENSION

a peek at your watch during sets to keep strict track of your intervals.

Weight selection is the key to an optimal Tabata training session. If the resistance is too light, overall training intensity will be insufficient and results inadequate. If the weight is too heavy, you won't be able to adhere to the 20-seconds-on, 10-seconds-off intervals for all eight sets. In this case, rest periods get bloated and you'll no longer reap the aerobic benefits of Tabata training.

It'll take some trial and error to select the proper

Because the Tabata program, as it's laid out here, is both painfully intense and high in volume — which anyone will agree is a brutal combination — we suggest you train each muscle group only once per week to provide for ample recovery. Follow the Tabata Interval Training program for 4–6 weeks before going back to more traditional straight-sets training. Return to Tabata only every 2–3 months. Trust us, the program's so demanding that you really won't want to come back more often than that.

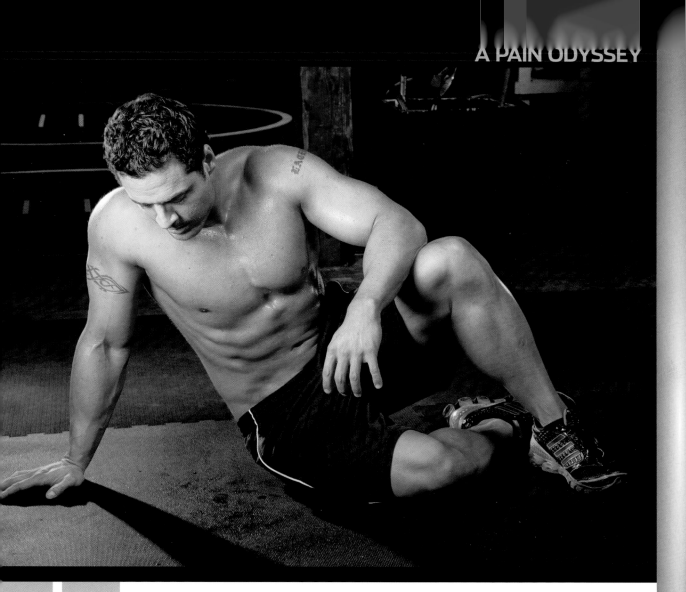

Brutally effective, Tabata Interval Training is so far out of the three-sets-of-10-reps box it doesn't even speak the same language

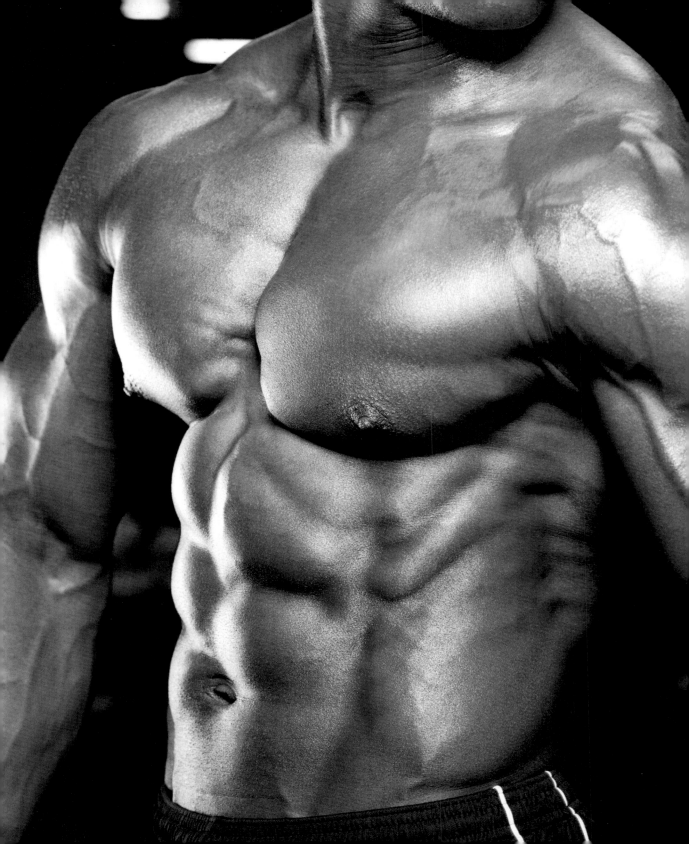

FULFILL YOUR DENSITY

BUILD MUSCLE AND BURN BODYFAT IN LESS TIME WITH THE INNOVATIVE EDT SYSTEM

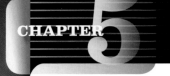
Hey — want to do something really different in the gym that won't take as long as those 30–40-set, train-to-failure-at-all-costs marathon sessions, yet will still make you bigger and leaner? These new workouts won't hurt as much as your standard forced reps, drop sets and rest-pauses, but you'll still train with plenty of intensity. In fact, experiencing less pain is kind of the point of Escalating Density Training (EDT) created by renowned strength coach Charles Staley, BS, MSS, director of Staley Training Systems in Gilbert, Arizona (staleytraining.com).

"A lot of people assess the value or productivity of a training session based on how much it hurts, and that's a mistake," Staley says. "Fitness is a result of what you do, not what you feel. The focus should be on the amount and quality of work accomplished. When you do EDT workouts you'll probably be hurting, but pain isn't the goal. If you're sore the next day, it's because you're emphasizing performance over pain."

Confused? Don't worry, it'll make sense soon. Here's how it works:

WHAT EDT IS

You select two exercises for opposing muscle groups (such as chest/back or legs/shoulders) and alternate sets between the two for 15 minutes. That's one PR (personal record) zone. Note how much weight you used and how many reps you performed for each exercise, and try to improve those numbers about a week later when you pair the same two exercises again. This helps you quantify how much work you've done. If the next time out you do more reps of each exercise with the same weight in the same 15-minute period, you've set a new PR and the workout was a success. EDT workouts are measurable and objective, and that's a good thing.

WHAT IT DOES

EDT routines are designed to improve body composition — helping you build muscle and lose bodyfat via intense (if relatively brief) training sessions. EDT can also be used to get stronger; simply increase the resistance and decrease the reps. But can you really get bigger, stronger and leaner in such a short time?

"There's no question," Staley says. "This system is all about altering body composition. EDT can make you bigger, leaner and stronger; it works quickly; and although you train hard, it's enjoyable because the workout is a competition with yourself. There's a cardio benefit as well."

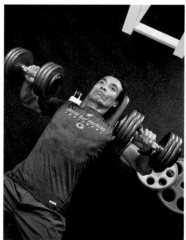
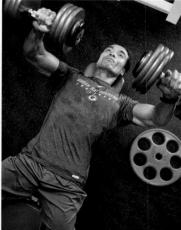
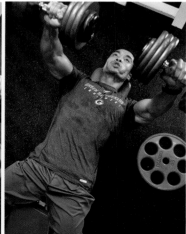

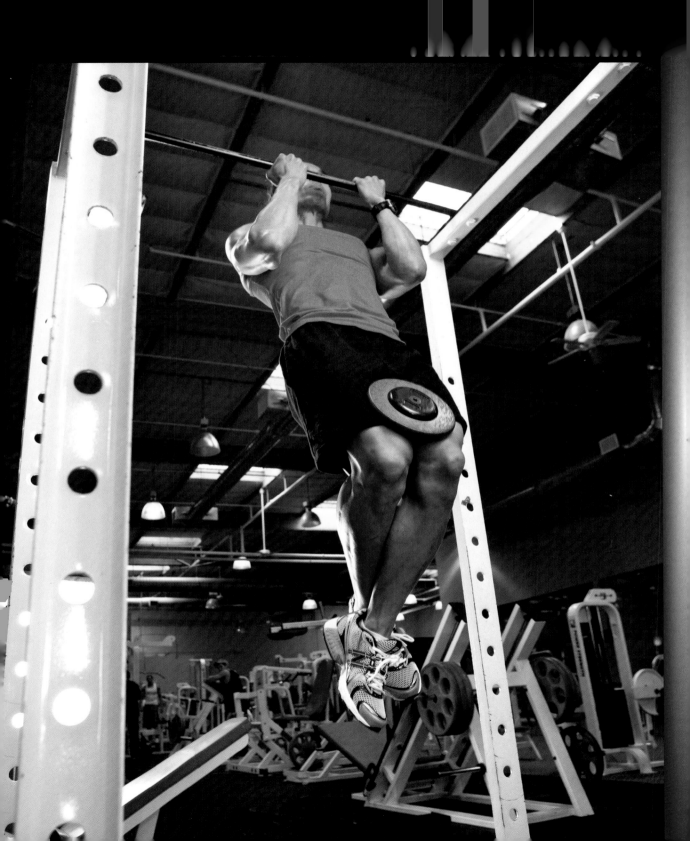

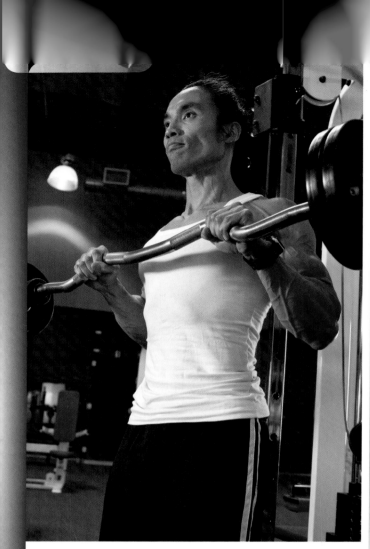

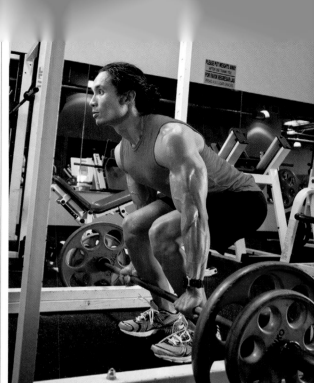

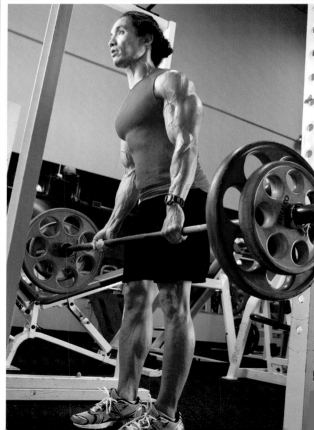

WHAT EDT IS NOT

EDT isn't about training to failure, at least not until the very end of a PR zone. If you select a weight for an exercise that's your 10-rep max (RM), for example, you'll do no more than five reps at a time. At least early on in the 15 minutes, this will have you stopping well short of failure.

"If you pace yourself — which in this case means not going to failure — you'll be able to do more work, and a big component of hypertrophy is the mechanical work performed," Staley explains. "If you train to failure on the first set, you drastically limit how much work you can continue to do. That said, it's okay to train to failure at the end of a PR zone."

EDT PROGRAM

Below is a sample four-day-split, 12-week EDT program. Within each four-week phase, exercise pairings (PR zones) are repeated once a week. Each workout includes one required ("compulsory") PR zone and one optional PR zone, each lasting 15 minutes, not including warm-ups. Whether you should complete the optional zone depends on your experience and fatigue level. Beginners should start with only the compulsory zone; advanced lifters can do both, but should forgo the optional zone if overtraining is evident.

The program is designed to work different bodyparts every four weeks to promote muscular balance and provide rest for potentially overstressed areas. For example, in Weeks 1–4, the shoulders are involved in every workout (chest/back and legs/shoulders PR zones), which could lead to overtraining. So direct shoulder work is minimized in Weeks 5–8, then reintroduced in Weeks 9–12.

>> For each PR zone, the resistance is listed in parentheses — from 6RM–20RM — to target size, strength and endurance, and also enhance fat-burning, over the course of 12 weeks. Always start with half the RM. When 10RM is indicated, start with five reps; when 20RM is indicated, reps start at 10.

>> Within each PR zone, alternate between the two exercises, resting as needed, for 15 minutes. Record the total reps performed for each exercise — that's your PR, which you'll attempt to beat next time out.

WEEKS 1–4

DAY 1
Compulsory: Dip/Pull-Up* (10RM)
Optional: Hammer Curl/Lying Triceps Extension (20RM)

DAY 2
Compulsory: Front Squat/ Barbell Push Press (10RM)
Optional: Back Extension/ Hanging Leg Raise (20RM)

DAY 3
Compulsory: Incline Dumbbell Press/Seated Cable Row (10RM)
Optional: Barbell Curl/ Pushdown (20RM)

DAY 4
Compulsory: Deadlift/ Dumbbell Front Raise (10RM)
Optional: Step-Up (right leg)/ Step-Up (left leg) (20RM)

WEEKS 5–8

DAY 1
Compulsory: Front Squat/ Seated Cable Row (10RM)
Optional: Standing Calf Raise/ Barbell Shrug (20RM)

DAY 2
Compulsory: Dumbbell Bench Press/Hammer Curl (10RM)
Optional: Lying Triceps Extension/Reverse Curl (20RM)

DAY 3
Compulsory: Deadlift/ Chin (10RM)
Optional: Exercise-Ball Crunch/ Lateral Raise (20RM)

DAY 4
Compulsory: Dip/Barbell Curl (10RM)
Optional: Back Extension/ Push-Up (20RM)

WEEKS 9–12

DAY 1
Compulsory: Chin/Front Squat (6RM)
Optional: Hammer Curl/ Standing Calf Raise (16RM)

DAY 2
Compulsory: Dumbbell Overhead Press/Seated Cable Row (10RM)
Optional: Reverse Curl/ Cable Crunch (16RM)

DAY 3
Compulsory: Dumbbell Bench Press/Squat (10RM)
Optional: Dumbbell Lying Triceps Extension/Barbell Shrug (16RM)

DAY 4
Compulsory: Pull-Up/Push-Up (8RM)
Optional: Lunge (right leg)/ Lunge (left leg) (12RM)

* If you can do more than 10 reps of dips or pull-ups, add weight; if you can't do 10 dips or pull-ups, use an assisted dip/pull-up machine.

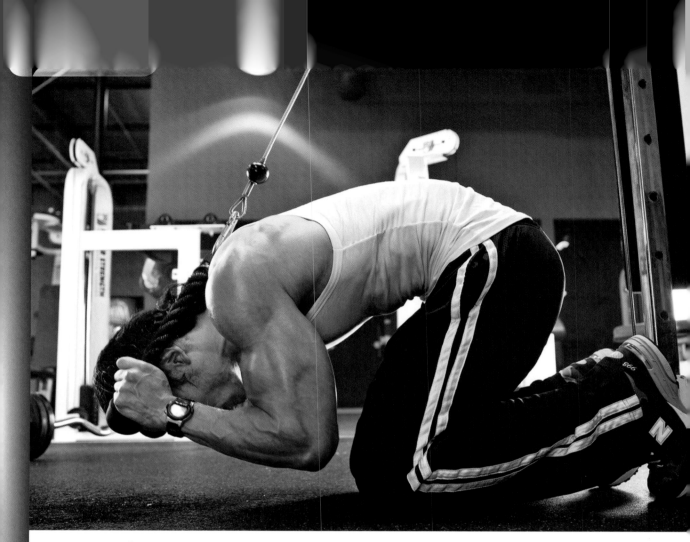

Early on in a PR zone, you might rest only 5–10 seconds between exercises, but as you near the 15-minute cutoff, those rest periods may reach one minute. "As fatigue accumulates, you'll want to throw some longer rest periods in there," Staley says. "Be sure your form is good throughout. The beauty of EDT is that you make your own decisions; you have to learn the best way to pace yourself."

HOW TO DO IT

Here's how you'll perform each PR zone:

» **Select two exercises from opposing muscle groups.** They don't have to be exact antagonists such as chest/back, biceps/triceps, quads/hamstrings or abs/lower back; you can also pair leg and shoulder exercises or quad and bi's moves. What's important is that you make sure each exercise fatigues only one muscle group. If you paired an incline press with a military press, for example, your delts would get so fried that you probably couldn't complete the 15 minutes.

» **Select an equivalent resistance for each exercise,** from heavy (4RM) to moderate (10–12RM) to light (40+RM), depending on whether you want to focus on strength, size or endurance. Whatever resistance/RM you select, start off doing half that number of reps. For example, if you go with your 10RM on incline presses and lat pulldowns, begin with five reps of each.

» Start your stopwatch. Using a 10RM on incline presses and pulldowns as an example, do five reps of inclines, rest as needed (which will be very brief early on) and then do five reps of pulldowns. Continue in this manner until five reps is too much, then drop to four reps of each exercise. When four reps becomes too difficult, drop to three, and so on. By the end of the PR zone, you may still be doing five reps or alternating exercises every rep. When your stopwatch hits 15 minutes, that PR zone is over. Record your weight and total reps. A typical PR zone might look like this: 6x5, 3x4, 3x3, 3x2, 2x1, for 59 total reps per exercise. That's your current PR for that exercise pairing.

» About one week later, do the same two exercises, using the same weight as before, and try to do more than 59 reps to set a new PR. It doesn't matter how you reach your new PR; you can do more sets of five early on or do more sets of three in the middle.

"There's no wrong or right way to do this," Staley says. "The end justifies the means, and I'm not terribly concerned with the sets and reps. The focus should be on how much work is accomplished in that 15 minutes."

HOW TO PROGRESS

The point of EDT is to increase the amount of work you can do within a set period. In other words, it's all about making progress. Simply doing more reps with the same weight will allow you to progress, but soon enough you'll need (and want) to add weight.

Staley has a simple formula for determining when to increase resistance: the 20/5 Rule. Once you exceed your baseline PR — the number of reps you did the first time you performed the exercise — by 20% or more, increase the load by 5% or 5 pounds, whichever is less. It might take you 2–3 repeats to be ready to increase the weight or you might want to up the resistance on your

second go-around. Either way, once you add weight, you'll wipe the slate clean and build from that point.

If you don't beat your PR, the 20/5 Rule works in reverse: If the number of reps performed is 20% less than your current PR, *reduce* your weight by 5% or 5 pounds (whichever is more) the next time out.

"Good performance, which is an indicator that you've fully recovered, is rewarded by heavier loads," Staley says. "Poor performance, however, means you haven't recovered, so you'll lift lighter loads as a form of active recovery. This reasoning runs counter to most people's intuition. But if you're weak, you need time to recover, not greater volume."

HOW OFTEN TO DO IT

To make significant improvements on your PRs, perform a given exercise pairing weekly for at least 3–4 weeks before changing the movements. But keep in mind: If you lift four days a week, you'll pair different exercises each workout. (See the sample program on page 55.) Let's say on Monday you paired incline presses and lat pulldowns. On Thursday you'd do chest and back again, but with two different moves, perhaps dips and pull-ups. In this case, you'd do each exercise pairing only once a week.

HOW TO TWEAK EDT

There's a lot of flexibility in EDT, despite the finite lifting periods. But there's a reason each PR zone is only 15 minutes. "I believe more than that is excessive," Staley says. "I also believe in putting a time limit on your training. That's one of the best ways to get work done. But I'm not against people getting creative with my suggestions. If you want to experiment with longer or shorter PR zones or [more workouts per week], I'm fine with that. Just try it my way before you make any modifications."

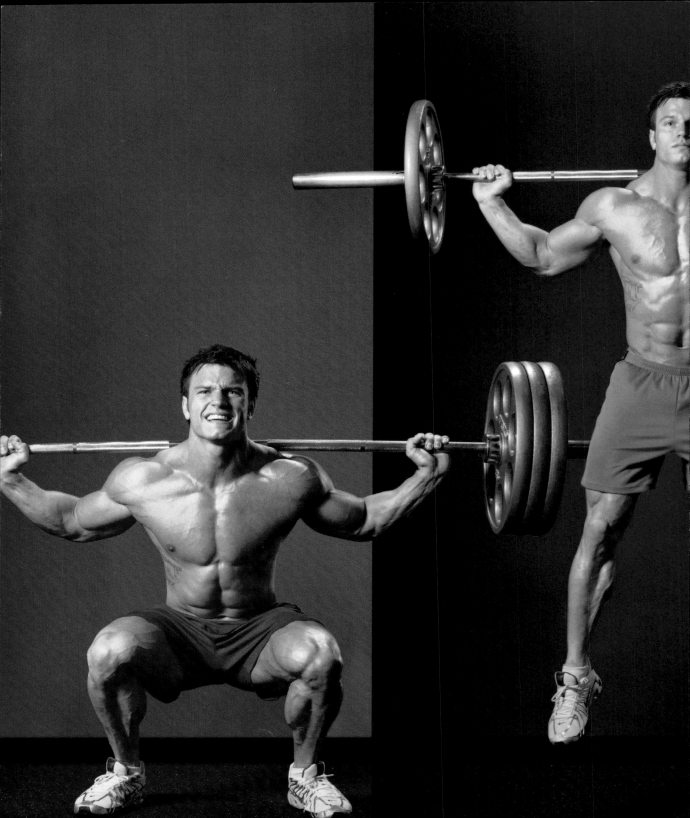

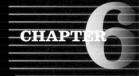
THE STRENGTH AND POWER COMPLEX

THIS SIX-WEEK TRAINING PROTOCOL SHOWS YOU HOW TO ACHIEVE IMMEDIATE STRENGTH AND POWER FOR LONG-TERM GAINS

power : (pouʹər)

-*noun* 1. energy, force or momentum : with speed
Power = force *x* velocity

We all know guys who seem to have spent most of their adult lives wrestling with one complex after another, moving from a Peter Pan to an Oedipus to a Napoleon Complex before succumbing to the warm embrace of an Inferiority Complex. You've probably seen them in the gym, fingering the heavy weights before slinking back into the rows of Nautilus machines to be lost forever. That's what we call the Castration Complex.

But here at M&F we deal with success stories, and our job is to even the playing field so everyone — even those with an Electra Complex — can achieve measurable results. To that end, we've

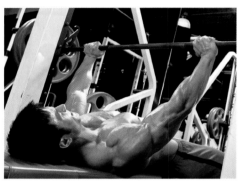

come up with a program that provides immediate gains in power and strength that must be maintained over time to be effective, but immediate power-and-strength gratification nonetheless.

The program is called Complex Training and it works like this: You do two similar exercises with two extreme weight amounts — one very heavy, one very light — to boost your performance on the second move. In theory, it runs counter to the prevailing practice of doing your hardest exercise first. By following this program you'll increase strength or explosive power on the *second* exercise, depending on how you order the moves.

M&F POWER AND SPEED COMPLEX | WEEKS 1, 3, 5

›› When performing the Power and Speed Complex, use a weight for the first exercise with which you can do only five reps, rest for five minutes, then perform the explosive exercise for three reps. Rest three minutes and repeat this sequence twice more. Choose one exercise from each column for each muscle group to perform at the beginning of your regular workout for that bodypart.

MUSCLE GROUP	EXERCISE 1	EXERCISE 2
CHEST	Smith Machine Bench Press Bench Press	Smith Machine Brench-Press Throw Power Push-Up
SHOULDERS	Smith Machine Shoulder Press Barbell Shoulder Press	Smith Machine Shoulder-Press Throw Medicine-Ball Overhead Throw
BACK	Smith Machine One-Arm Row One-Arm Dumbbell Row	Smith Machine One-Arm Power Row
LEGS	Squat Smith Machine Squat	Jump Squat Vertical Jump Sprint

COMPLEX TRAINING

Complex Training is most effective at the beginning of your workout. On chest day, for example, start with Complex bench presses and push presses, then continue with a typical chest workout. Although postactivation potentiation is an acute phenomenon, it can enhance strength, power and speed over the course of the program. Alternate the order of the exercise complexes (light/heavy, heavy/light) every week until you complete three cycles. This way you build strength and power, which is the best way to boost overall performance whether your goals are gym-based or sport-specific.

WORKOUT 1 — MONDAY: CHEST, TRICEPS, ABS

MUSCLE GROUP	EXERCISE	SETS/REPS	REST
CHEST	Smith Machine Bench Press	1/5	5 min.
	Smith Machine Bench-Press Throw[1]	1/3	3 min.
	Smith Machine Bench Press	1/5	5 min.
	Smith Machine Bench-Press Throw[1]	1/3	3 min.
	Smith Machine Bench Press	1/5	5 min.
	Smith Machine Bench-Press Throw[1]	1/3	3 min.
	Incline Dumbbell Press	3/8–10	2–3 min.
	Cable Crossover	3/8–10	1–2 min.
TRICEPS	Close-Grip Bench Press	3/8–10	2–3 min.
	Pressdown	3/8–10	2–3 min.
ABS	Reverse Crunch — superset with —	3/to failure	—
	Crunch	3/to failure	1–2 min.

[1] Use a weight equivalent to 30%–50% of your 1RM on the bench press.

WORKOUT 2 — TUESDAY: LEGS, CALVES

MUSCLE GROUP	EXERCISE	SETS/REPS	REST
LEGS	Squat	1/5	5 min.
	Jump Squat[1]	1/3	3 min.
	Squat	1/5	5 min.
	Jump Squat[1]	1/3	3 min.
	Squat	1/5	5 min.
	Jump Squat[1]	1/3	3 min.
	Leg Press	3/8–10	2–3 min.
	Leg Extension	2/8–10	1–2 min.
	Romanian Deadlift	2/8–10	2–3 min.
	Lying Leg Curl	2/8–10	1–2 min.
CALVES	Standing Calf Raise — superset with —	3/12–15	—
	Seated Calf Raise	3/15–20	1–2 min.

[1] Use your bodyweight or a weight equivalent to 30% of your 1RM on the squat.

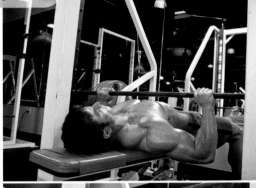

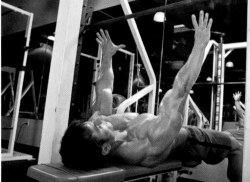

SMITH MACHINE
BENCH-PRESS THROW
>> Start with the racked bar at full arm extension and positioned over your lower chest. Using a shoulder-width or slightly wider grip, unrack and lower the bar, keeping your elbows out to your sides. Touch your chest with the bar, pause, then press back up explosively so the bar leaves your hands. Absorb the descent smoothly.

If you want to boost your strength on the bench press, for example, first do a bench-press-type exercise, such as a bench-press throw or power push-up with very light weight, rest five minutes, then perform the bench press. You'll be noticeably stronger. On the flip side, if you want to increase explosive power on the bench press, first do the bench press with a very heavy weight (90%–95% of your one-rep max), rest five minutes, then do the bench-press throw or power push-up with very light weight. You'll have significantly more power.

JUMP SQUAT
>> Get in the same starting position as a regular squat. Using a faster-than-usual descent, squat down until your thighs are parallel to the floor. Without pausing, extend your knees and hips explosively and try to jump as high as possible. Absorb the landing by bending your knees, and set up for the next rep.

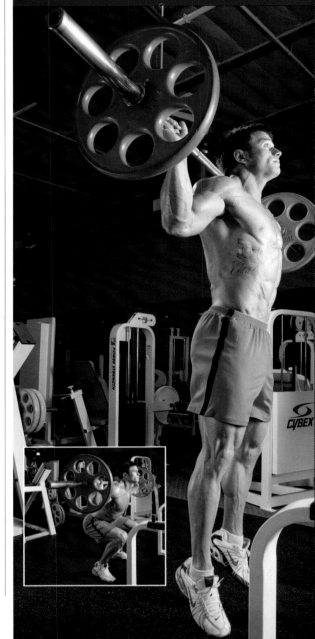

HIGHER GROUND

This graph shows the percent increase in jump height and force when test subjects performed the vertical jump after completing one set of five reps of the squat or power clean compared to jumping after a typical warm-up. Above the waist, postactivation potentiation results follow a similar pattern. A recent study from the University of Zagreb (Croatia) had trained subjects perform a seated medicine-ball throw with a 9-pound ball after a normal warm-up. The subjects also did one set of three reps of the bench press using their three-rep max, rested for three minutes, then did the medicine-ball throw. When subjects performed the bench press first, they threw the medicine ball more than 8% faster than after the basic warm-up.

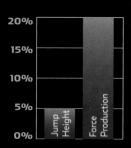

WORKOUT 3 — THURSDAY: SHOULDERS, TRAPS, ABS

MUSCLE GROUP	EXERCISE	SETS/REPS	REST
SHOULDERS	Barbell Shoulder Press	1/5	5 min.
	Medicine-Ball Overhead Throw[1]	1/3	3 min.
	Barbell Shoulder Press	1/5	5 min.
	Medicine-Ball Overhead Throw[1]	1/3	3 min.
	Barbell Shoulder Press	1/5	5 min.
	Medicine-Ball Overhead Throw[1]	1/3	3 min.
	Smith Machine Upright Row	3/8–10	2–3 min.
	Bent-Over Lateral Raise	3/8–10	1–2 min.
TRAPS	Barbell Shrug	4/8–10	2–3 min.
ABS	Hanging Leg Raise	3/to failure	—
	— superset with —		
	Cable Crunch	3/8–10	1–2 min.

[1] Use an 8–20-pound medicine ball.

WORKOUT 4 — FRIDAY: BACK, BICEPS, FOREARMS

MUSCLE GROUP	EXERCISE	SETS/REPS	REST
BACK	Smith Machine One-Arm Row	1/5	5 min.
	Smith Machine One-Arm Power Row	1/3	3 min.
	Smith Machine One-Arm Row	1/5	5 min.
	Smith Machine One-Arm Power Row	1/3	3 min.
	Smith Machine One-Arm Row	1/5	5 min.
	Smith Machine One-Arm Power Row	1/3	3 min.
	Lat Pulldown	3/8–10	2–3 min.
	Seated Cable Row	2/8–10	2–3 min.
BICEPS	Barbell Curl	3/8–10	2–3 min.
	Incline Dumbbell Curl	3/8–10	2–3 min.
FOREARMS	Barbell Wrist Curl	3/8–10	1–2 min.

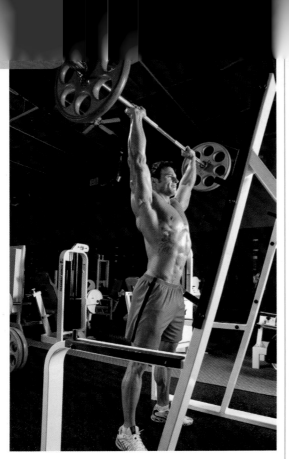

Scientifically, Complex Training involves the phenomenon of postactivation potentiation, the idea that the first exercise boosts the number of muscle fibers used in the second exercise, thereby enhancing strength and power. The precise mechanism at work isn't entirely known, but a few theories exist. One based on the nervous system maintains that the first exercise ramps up the nerves that stimulate the muscle fibers to contract, causing faster and more synchronous nerve firing, which results in greater power and strength in those fibers.

Another theory suggests that the first exercise enhances the biochemistry of the muscle fibers, basically priming them to contract with more power and force. Whether one or both of these theories are at play in Complex Training, the bottom line is it works. And beyond the power and strength gains you'll make, prepare yourself for a little Superiority Complex. Who couldn't use a bit of that from time to time?

BARBELL
SHOULDER PRESS
>> Stand erect with your feet shoulder-width apart and take a wider than shoulder-width grip on the bar racked at upper-chest level. Unrack the weight and press it straight up, keeping your core tight and head neutral. When your elbows near full extension, pause and return the bar to your chest. The explosive/plyometric version of this exercise is the Smith machine shoulder-press throw (not pictured), performed in the same manner as the Smith bench-press throw, only overhead.

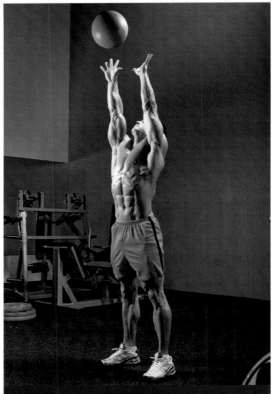

MEDICINE-BALL
OVERHEAD THROW
>> Hold the medicine ball at your chest with your elbows high, knees and hips bent, and feet shoulder-width apart. Simultaneously extend your knees and hips and drive the ball straight up as fast as you can. Note: Do not attempt to catch the ball.

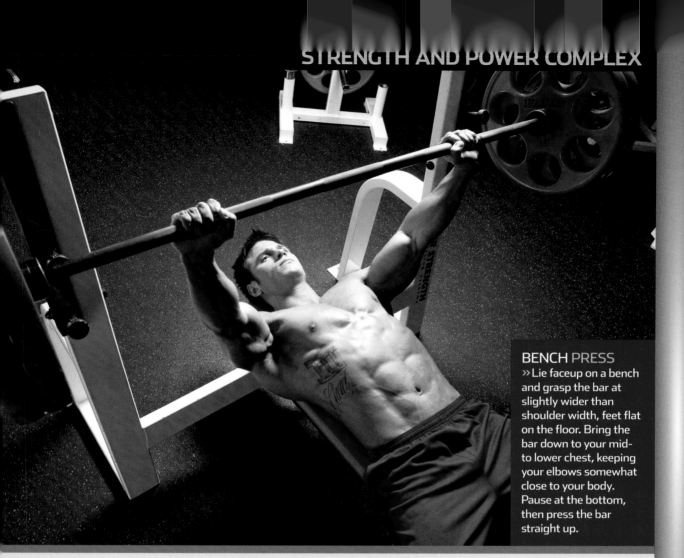

BENCH PRESS
>> Lie faceup on a bench and grasp the bar at slightly wider than shoulder width, feet flat on the floor. Bring the bar down to your mid- to lower chest, keeping your elbows somewhat close to your body. Pause at the bottom, then press the bar straight up.

M&F STRENGTH COMPLEX | WEEKS 2, 4, 6

>> When performing the Strength Complex, do three reps of a plyometric-style or explosive exercise like plyometric push-ups, rest 30–60 seconds, then do a one-rep-max set. Choose one exercise from each column for each muscle group to perform at the beginning of your regular workout for that bodypart.

MUSCLE GROUP	EXERCISE 1	EXERCISE 2
CHEST	Plyometric Push-Up Power Push-Up Smith Machine Bench-Press Throw	Bench Press
SHOULDERS	Smith Machine Shoulder-Press Throw Medicine-Ball Overhead Throw	Barbell Shoulder Press
BACK	Smith Machine One-Arm Power Row	Smith Machine One-Arm Row One-Arm Dumbbell Row
LEGS	Depth Jump Jump Squat	Squat

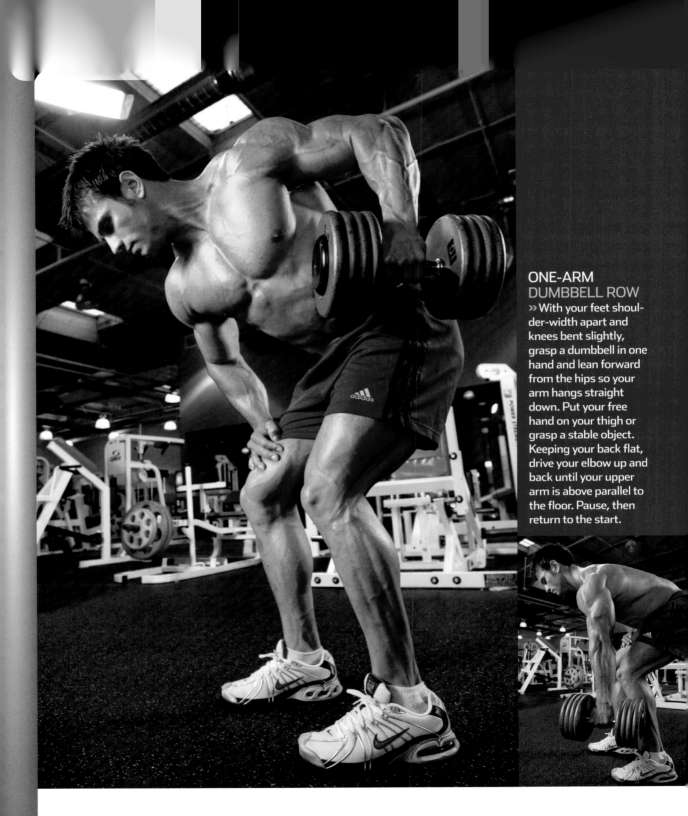

ONE-ARM
DUBBELL ROW

» With your feet shoulder-width apart and knees bent slightly, grasp a dumbbell in one hand and lean forward from the hips so your arm hangs straight down. Put your free hand on your thigh or grasp a stable object. Keeping your back flat, drive your elbow up and back until your upper arm is above parallel to the floor. Pause, then return to the start.

WORKOUT 1 — MONDAY: CHEST, TRICEPS, ABS

MUSCLE GROUP	EXERCISE	SETS/REPS	REST
CHEST	Plyometric Push-Up[1]	1/3	30–60 sec.
	Bench Press	1/1	2–3 min.
	Bench Press	3/6–8	2–3 min.
	Incline Bench Press	3/6–8	2–3 min.
TRICEPS	Close-Grip Bench Press	3/6–8	2–3 min.
	Dumbbell Overhead Extension	3/6–8	2–3 min.
ABS	Reverse Crunch	3/to failure	—
	— superset with —		
	Crunch	3/to failure	1–2 min.

[1] First perform 2–3 warm-up sets of the bench press, progressing in weight until you reach about 75% of your 1RM on the last warm-up set.

WORKOUT 2 — TUESDAY: LEGS, CALVES

MUSCLE GROUP	EXERCISE	SETS/REPS	REST
LEGS	Depth Jump[1]	1/3	30–60 sec.
	Squat	1/1	2–3 min.
	Squat	3/6–8	2–3 min.
	Leg Extension	2/8–10	1–2 min.
	Romanian Deadlift	2/6–8	2–3 min.
	Lying Leg Curl	2/8–10	1–2 min.
CALVES	Standing Calf Raise	3/10–12	—
	— superset with —		
	Seated Calf Raise	3/12–15	1–2 min.

[1] First perform 2–3 warm-up sets of the squat, progressing in weight until you reach about 75% of your 1RM on the last warm-up set.

ɪgth : (strêngkth)

ʻorce: output required of one object to ʻother; Force = mass x acceleration

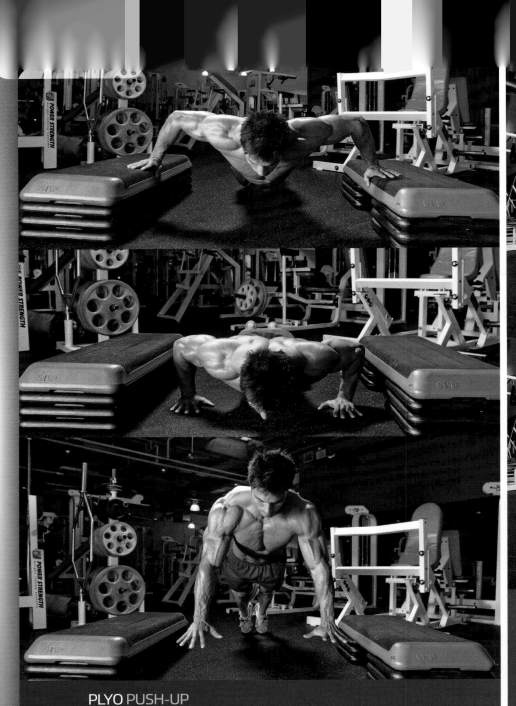

PLYO PUSH-UP

>> Place two blocks or steps parallel, then position yourself between them with your hands on top and your feet together on the floor. Drop down off the steps, bringing your hands under your shoulders in push-up position. Absorb the landing with your elbows and shoulders. Without pausing, drive up as hard as you can to push your upper body off the floor.

SMITH MACHINE
ONE-ARM
POWER ROW

>> With your feet shoul
width apart, right hand
your thigh and your to
about a 45-degree ang
grasp the bar at shin le
Quickly drive your left
back and up, releasing
bar when your upper a
comes parallel to the fl

STRONG RESULTS

This graph shows the increase in one-rep max (1RM) squat strength when test subjects performed depth jumps before squats compared to when they did a typical warm-up first. Researchers from the University of Massachusetts (Boston) tested athletes' squat 1RMs after doing a basic warm-up vs. three plyometric-style depth jumps from a 17-inch-high box. They found that subjects' average 1RM was about 300 pounds after the typical warm-up, but it increased to 310 pounds after they did the depth jumps.

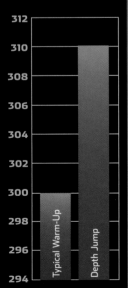

WORKOUT 3 — THURSDAY: SHOULDERS, TRAPS, ABS

MUSCLE GROUP	EXERCISE	SETS/REPS	REST
SHOULDERS	Medicine-Ball Overhead Throw[1,2]	1/3	30–60 sec.
	Barbell Shoulder Press	1/1	2–3 min.
	Barbell Shoulder Press	3/6–8	2–3 min.
	Barbell Upright Row	3/6–8	2–3 min.
	Bent-Over Lateral Raise	3/8–10	1–2 min.
TRAPS	Barbell Shrug	4/6–8	2–3 min.
ABS	Hanging Leg Raise — superset with —	3/to failure	—
	Cable Crunch	3/8–10	1–2 min.

[1] Use an 8–20-pound medicine ball.
[2] First perform 2–3 warm-up sets of the barbell shoulder press, progressing in weight until you reach about 75% of your 1RM on the last warm-up set.

WORKOUT 4 — FRIDAY: BACK, BICEPS, FOREARMS

MUSCLE GROUP	EXERCISE	SETS/REPS	REST
BACK	Smith Machine One-Arm Power Row[1]	1/3	30–60 sec.
	One-Arm Dumbbell Row	1/1	2–3 min.
	One-Arm Dumbbell Row	3/6–8	2–3 min.
	Lat Pulldown	3/6–8	2–3 min.
	Seated Cable Row	2/6–8	2–3 min.
BICEPS	Barbell Curl	3/6–8	2–3 min.
	Incline Dumbbell Curl	3/8–10	2–3 min.
FOREARMS	Barbell Wrist Curl	3/8–10	1–2 min.

[1] First perform 2–3 warm-up sets of the one-arm dumbbell row, progressing in weight until you reach about 75% of your 1RM on the last warm-up set.

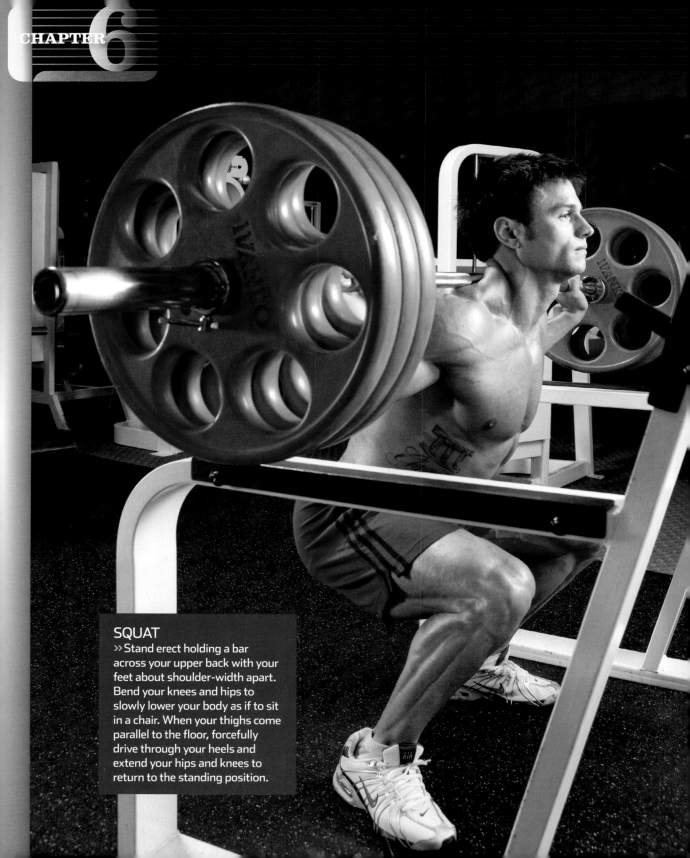

SQUAT

>> Stand erect holding a bar across your upper back with your feet about shoulder-width apart. Bend your knees and hips to slowly lower your body as if to sit in a chair. When your thighs come parallel to the floor, forcefully drive through your heels and extend your hips and knees to return to the standing position.

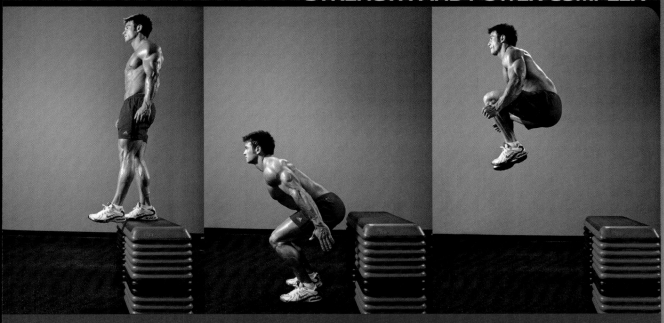

DEPTH JUMP

>> Step off a tall platform — do not jump — and absorb the landing with your hips and knees as you descend into a squat with your back flat and arms at your sides. Immediately drive through your lower body (hips, knees, ankles) to achieve as much height as possible.

MORE COMPLEX STUDIES THE TRUTH IS IN THE RESEARCH

If you're skeptical about our immediate-results claim, consider the numerous studies that have found this to be true. Australian researchers from the University of Ballarat (Victoria, Australia) performed one of the first studies on Complex Training. They reported in a 1998 issue of the *Journal of Strength & Conditioning Research* that when trained subjects performed five reps of squats using their five-rep max, rested for four minutes and did a jump squat on the Smith machine, they jumped 1.1 centimeters higher (a 3% increase in jump height) than when they didn't precede the jump squat with a set of heavy squats.

A 2001 study from the University of Memphis (Tennessee) found that when subjects performed 10 one-rep sets of the squat using 90% of their one-rep maxes (1RM, resting two minutes between sets) five minutes before a sprint test on a stationary cycle, they had 4% more power on the sprint test than when they performed the sprints without first doing the squats.

Moreover, University of Southern California (Los Angeles) researchers found equally compelling evidence for Complex Training. They reported in a 2003 issue of the *Journal of Strength & Conditioning Research* that when competitive athletes performed five one-rep sets of the squat using 90% of their 1RMs (resting two minutes between sets) five minutes before jump squats, they exhibited significantly more power and force than when they did the jump squats without first doing the squats.

More recently, researchers at East Stroudsburg University (Pennsylvania) tested athletes to see if Complex Training could lead to faster sprint times. They reported in a 2008 issue of the *Journal of Strength & Conditioning Research* that when test subjects did one three-rep set of squats using 70% of their 1RMs four minutes before sprinting, their average sprint speed was about 0.5 mph faster in the 40-meter sprint than when they didn't squat first. In a study presented at the 2008 Annual Meeting of the National Strength and Conditioning Association, researchers reported that athletes increased their vertical jump heights by more than 5% and force production by almost 20% when they performed a five-rep set of squats or power cleans using their five-rep max 4–5 minutes before performing the vertical jump compared to when they didn't do the five-rep set.

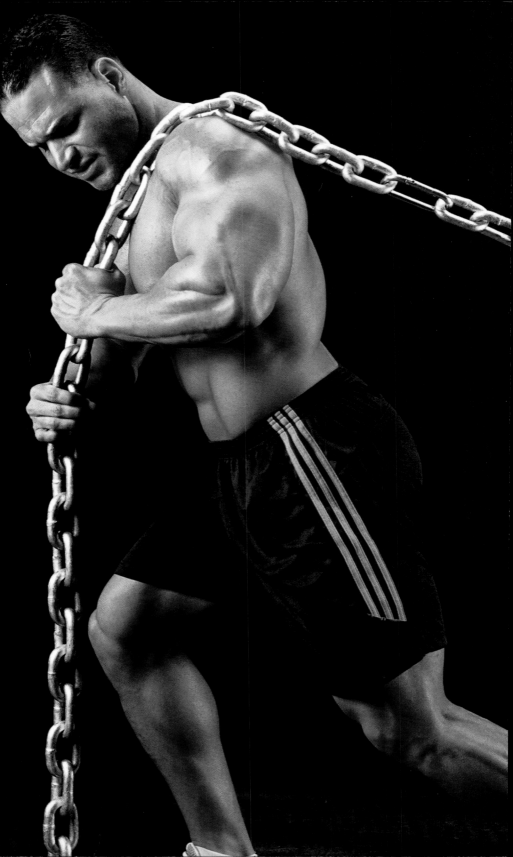

CHAIN
REACTION

BODYBUILDERS ARE JUST CATCHING ON TO WHAT POWERLIFTERS AND ELITE ATHLETES HAVE KNOWN FOR YEARS — THAT BANDS AND CHAINS CAN HELP YOU BUILD STRENGTH AND HEAPS OF DENSE, QUALITY MUSCLE

Weight belts, chalk, straps and truckloads of iron. For decades, these items have served as the basic equipment for building not only mounds of muscle but also raw, bar-bending strength. Over the years, these primitive implements have helped push the limits of the human physique, making it possible to win the battle against gravity day in and day out. But their most important contribution may be to one of the most basic mandates of weight-lifting: progressive overload.

The principle of progressive overload simply states that an increase in volume and intensity is required to achieve a targeted goal. Weight begets weight, and each workout is a step toward your objective. Bench-pressing 405 pounds one time, for example, requires a lifter to work his way up from his starting one-rep max with incrementally heavier loads until he reaches that 405-pound benchmark. How long it takes to reach a given goal is, of course, unique to each lifter. It could conceivably take one person years to hit that standard, while another may land in the coveted four-plates-per-side promised land after only months of training.

What about achieving progressive overload with each rep? Imagine the benefits you could reap from repetitions that get harder and heavier with each inch the weight is moved — challenging reps that offer no rest for muscles accustomed to recovering during lockouts or benefiting from elasticity. Weight belts, chalk, straps and truckloads of iron — they build muscle, all right. But to these things we now add chains and bands.

THE FUTURE OF STRENGTH?

The secret to both chains and bands is that they provide what's known as linear variable resistance. Linear variable resistance training (LVRT) refers to progressively increasing the resistance with the range of motion. Using the bench press as an example, the weight gets progressively heavier the farther you press the bar toward full arm extension. The increased resistance necessitates the

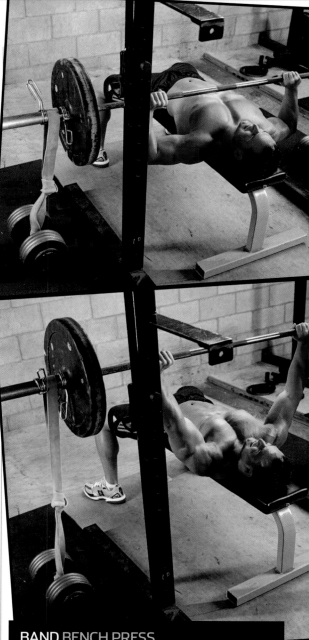

BAND BENCH PRESS
» When bench-pressing with bands, you can use heavy dumbbells to anchor them (see above) or loop them around the base of a power rack. Be sure to fix collars on the ends of the bar to hold the bands securely in place. Aim to generate maximum force on the positive rep.

BENCH PRESS Band Program

WEEK 1

EXERCISE	WEIGHT	%1RM	SETS/REPS
Bench Press	Band / Free weight / Total	10% / 20% / 30%	3/3-5
Bench Press	Free weight	70%	3/8-10
Incline Bench Press	-	-	3/10-12
Dumbbell Flye	-	-	3/10-12

WEEK 2

EXERCISE	WEIGHT	%1RM	SETS/REPS
Bench Press	Band / Free weight / Total	15% / 25% / 40%	3/3-5
Bench Press	Free weight	75%	3/8
Incline Bench Press	-	-	3/10
Dumbbell Flye	-	-	3/10

WEEK 3

EXERCISE	WEIGHT	%1RM	SETS/REPS
Bench Press	Band / Free weight / Total	15% / 35% / 50%	3/3-5
Bench Press	Free weight	80%	3/6-8
Incline Bench Press	-	-	3/8-10
Dumbbell Flye	-	-	3/8-10

WEEK 4

EXERCISE	WEIGHT	%1RM	SETS/REPS
Bench Press	Band / Free weight / Total	20% / 40% / 60%	3/3-5
Bench Press	Free weight	85%	3/4-6
Incline Bench Press	-	-	3/8
Dumbbell Flye	-	-	3/8

WEEK 5

EXERCISE	WEIGHT	%1RM	SETS/REPS
Bench Press	Band / Free weight / Total	20% / 50% / 70%	3/3-5
Bench Press	Free weight	90%	3/2-4
Incline Bench Press	-	-	3/6-8
Dumbbell Flye	-	-	3/6-8

WEEK 6

EXERCISE	WEIGHT	%1RM	SETS/REPS
Bench Press	Band / Free weight / Total	20% / 60% / 80%	3/3-5
Bench Press	Free weight	95%	3/1-2
Incline Bench Press	-	-	3/6
Dumbbell Flye	-	-	3/6-8

ONE-REP MAX CALCULATOR

NO PARTNER TO HELP YOU TEST YOUR 1RM? FINDING YOUR 5RM IS JUST AS GOOD

Just in case you're afraid of getting a bar pinned across your neck on a one-rep max (1RM) test, we've got a pretty reliable alternative. Research shows that using a five-rep max (5RM) to determine your 1RM is about 99% accurate for upper-body exercises and 97% accurate for lower-body exercises. That's close enough. Not to mention, if you want to build muscle it's more important to be strong with a weight you can lift for several reps than for just one — you don't get bigger by doing singles.

To calculate your 1RM for an exercise, find a weight that permits you to get five, and only five, reps; you shouldn't be able to get a sixth rep on your own. Take each weight and use one of these equations to determine your 1RM for the particular exercise.

>> FOR UPPER-BODY EXERCISES
(5RM weight x 1.1307) + 0.6998 = 1RM
Example: If you bench 300 pounds for five reps, your 1RM would be (300 x 1.1307) + 0.6998 = 340 pounds.

>> FOR LOWER-BODY EXERCISES
(5RM weight x 1.09703) + 14.2546 = 1RM
Example: If you squat 400 pounds for five reps, your 1RM would be (400 x 1.09703) + 14.2546 = 453 pounds, or 455 pounds (rounded up).

application of more force toward the top of the lift.

So what's the benefit to you? More muscle, that's what. As the range of motion lengthens and the resistance increases, the number of muscle fibers being used in the exercising muscle increases as well. The more muscle fibers being used, the greater the adaptations in strength that can be achieved.

Bands also boost force during the negative part of a rep because they increase its speed. This means you have to apply more force to stop the weight at the bottom of the movement. Again, the more force you have to apply, the greater the sum of muscle fibers that are called into action.

Imagine the benefits you could reap from reps that get harder and heavier with each inch the weight is moved

BAND AID

Need more convincing? One study conducted at Truman State University (Kirksville, Missouri) found that athletes who included elastic-resistance bench-press training in their regimens had a significantly greater increase in bench-press strength and power compared to those who utilized only free-weight resistance.

Another study, from the University of Wisconsin, La Crosse, reported in a 2006 issue of *The Journal of Strength & Conditioning Research* that when athletes used elastic-band training in addition to free-weight training, they had significantly more leg power than when they used only free weights.

Research shows that when comparing the same

exercise performed with elastic bands vs. free weights, the amount of muscle fibers activated and the amount of force provided by the muscle fibers are similar. Studies also show that programs using elastic tubing, elastic bands and like devices by themselves increase muscle strength and size and decrease bodyfat in a manner comparable to free-weight training.

CHAIN GANG

As you've probably gathered by now, most of the research done on LVRT has used elastic-band equipment, a rehabilitative device and fitness tool for almost a century. Chains, on the other hand, are new implements in the weight room, and they provide similar benefits to bands. The major difference is in how they work.

Chains provide resistance through the weight of each link. As they hang off the bar and pool on the floor, the only extra weight they provide is from the links between the bar and the floor. As you lift the bar higher, more links come off the floor and add weight to the bar. Elastic bands, on the other hand, provide resistance by a restoring force, which attempts to move the two ends of each band back to their original resting positions when they're pulled farther apart. The more you pull the bands (such as at the top of the range of motion of a squat), the greater the resistance.

TOOLS OF THE TRADE

We're not telling you to use LVRT in place of free weights; we're telling you to consider using chains and bands *with* free weights. By increasing the amount of force it takes to move a weight from point A to point B, chains and bands can build denser, stronger muscles. And what bodybuilder wouldn't want that?

So how do you get chains and bands into the gym and use them? By picking up a set of each from suppliers such as elitefts.com and following our advice in "Banded & Chained."

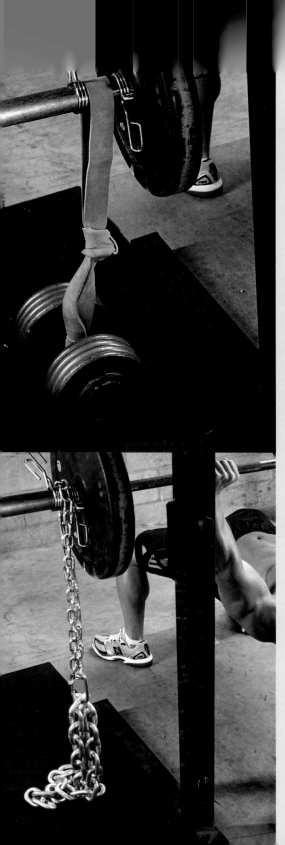

BANDED & CHAINED

You can perform many exercises with bands and chains, but the bench press and squat best capitalize on their vertical resistance

» Bands How you set up bands depends on the equipment you have available in your gym. Do your squats in a power rack. You can loop the bands around the bottom of the rack, or place the safety bars in the lowest position and loop the bands around them. Wrap the other end around the end of the bar. The bench press may also need to be performed in a power rack with the bands set up as suggested for the squat, or you can loop the bands around very heavy dumbbells. Regardless of how you set up your bands, be sure you do so properly and evenly. If not, one side may have more tension than the other and cause the bar to be uneven. See the photos at left for examples.

You'll need to know your one-rep max (1RM) to determine the amount of free-weight and band resistance to put on the bar. Do a true 1RM test under partner supervision or estimate it by using our 1RM formula (see "One-Rep Max Calculator" on page 75).

» Chains Setting up chains is a bit simpler than bands, but carrying the extra weight with you to the gym can be a clangy, awkward mess. But hey, if that's all you have to bear to add some new bulk, so be it. If you order the complete set of chains from elitefts.com, you'll get two $^3/_8$" chains and two $^5/_8$" chains. The $^3/_8$" chain is used to wrap around the end of the bar and hold the $^5/_8$" chain. One $^3/_8$" chain (5 pounds) plus one $^5/_8$" chain (20 pounds) weighs about 25 pounds. You may have to use additional chain weight depending on your strength.

When setting up the chains on the bar, it's crucial that the $^5/_8$" chains rest completely on the floor in the bottom position. For the squat, consider setting up the chains so that a few links still rest on the floor in the top position. This will prevent the chains from swinging, especially when you walk the bar out of the rack. For the bench press, only about half of the links will be off the floor in the top position due to the short range of motion. That means if you have one set each of $^3/_8$" chains and $^5/_8$" chains on the bar, you'll be using an additional 30 pounds of chain weight, not 50 pounds.

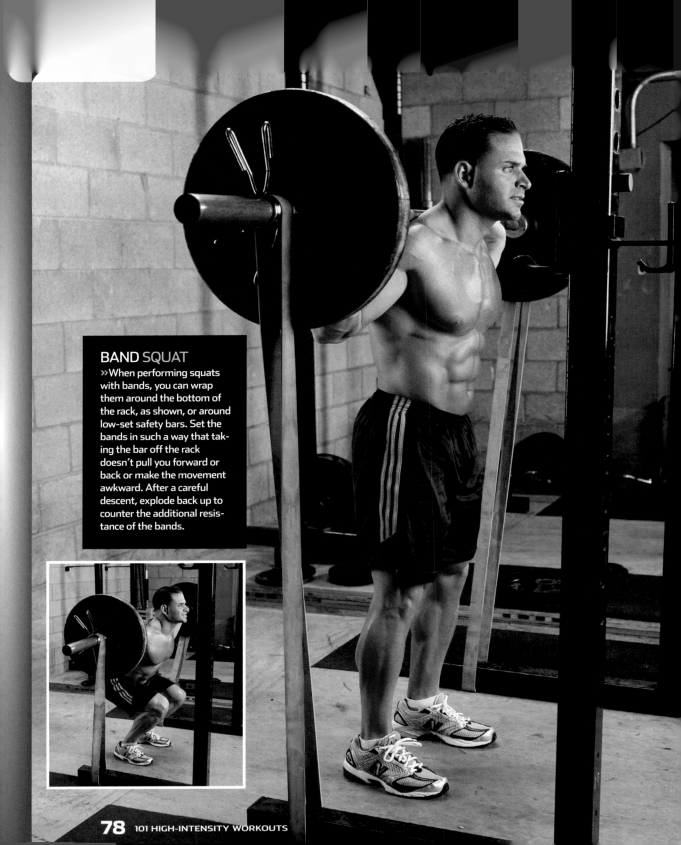

BAND SQUAT

»When performing squats with bands, you can wrap them around the bottom of the rack, as shown, or around low-set safety bars. Set the bands in such a way that taking the bar off the rack doesn't pull you forward or back or make the movement awkward. After a careful descent, explode back up to counter the additional resistance of the bands.

SQUAT Band Program

WEEK 1

EXERCISE	WEIGHT	%1RM	SETS/REPS
Squat	Band	10%	3/3–5
	Free weight	20%	
	Total	30%	
Squat	Free weight	70%	3/8–10
Leg Press	–	–	3/10–12
Leg Extension	–	–	3/10–12
Romanian Deadlift	–	–	3/10–12

WEEK 2

EXERCISE	WEIGHT	%1RM	SETS/REPS
Squat	Band	15%	3/3–5
	Free weight	25%	
	Total	40%	
Squat	Free weight	75%	3/8
Leg Press	–	–	3/10
Leg Extension	–	–	3/10
Romanian Deadlift	–	–	3/10

WEEK 3

EXERCISE	WEIGHT	%1RM	SETS/REPS
Squat	Band	15%	3/3–5
	Free weight	35%	
	Total	50%	
Squat	Free weight	80%	3/6–8
Leg Press	–	–	3/8–10
Leg Extension	–	–	3/8–10
Romanian Deadlift	–	–	3/8–10

WEEK 4

EXERCISE	WEIGHT	%1RM	SETS/REPS
Squat	Band	20%	3/3–5
	Free weight	40%	
	Total	60%	
Squat	Free weight	85%	3/4–6
Leg Press	–	–	3/8
Leg Extension	–	–	3/8
Romanian Deadlift	–	–	3/8

WEEK 5

EXERCISE	WEIGHT	%1RM	SETS/REPS
Squat	Band	20%	3/3–5
	Free weight	50%	
	Total	70%	
Squat	Free weight	90%	3/2–4
Leg Press	–	–	3/6–8
Leg Extension	–	–	3/6–8
Romanian Deadlift	–	–	3/6–8

WEEK 6

EXERCISE	WEIGHT	%1RM	SETS/REPS
Squat	Band	20%	3/3–5
	Free weight	60%	
	Total	80%	
Squat	Free weight	95%	3/1–2
Leg Press	–	–	3/6
Leg Extension	–	–	3/6–8
Romanian Deadlift	–	–	3/6–8

BAND RESISTANCE

To determine the resistance supplied by unmarked bands, stand on a scale holding an empty bar in the top position of a squat with the bands set up. Be sure to deduct your bodyweight and the weight of the bar (most Olympic bars are 45 pounds). If you get the band pack from Elite Fitness (elitefts.com), it supplies several different bands with the amounts of resistance specified. Find the one that provides the amount of resistance needed. In some cases, you may need to use more than one band to obtain the right resistance.

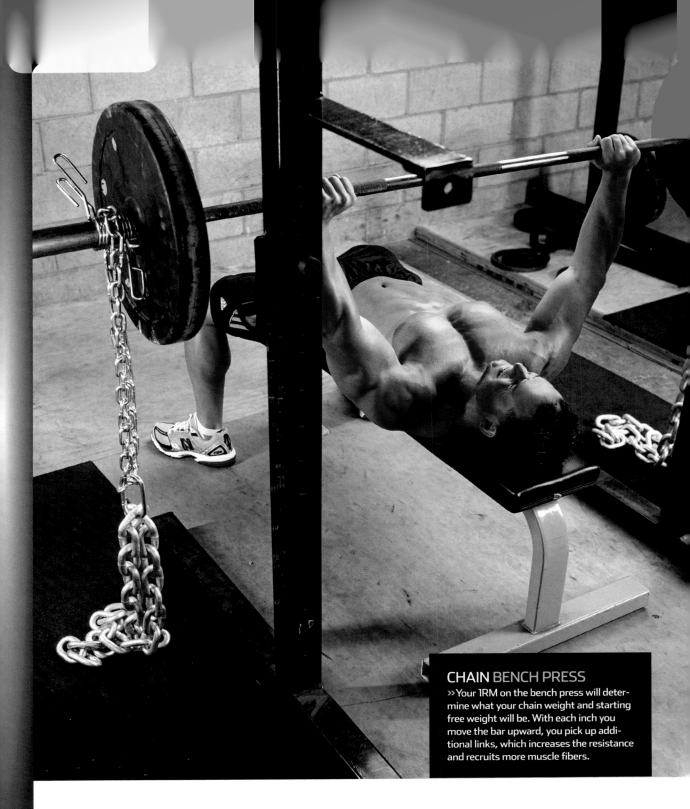

CHAIN BENCH PRESS

>> Your 1RM on the bench press will determine what your chain weight and starting free weight will be. With each inch you move the bar upward, you pick up additional links, which increases the resistance and recruits more muscle fibers.

BENCH PRESS Chain Program

FOR CHAIN WEIGHT, SEE "OFF THE CHAIN" TO DETERMINE HOW MUCH RESISTANCE TO USE.
REMEMBER, ON BENCH PRESSES YOU'RE USING ONLY HALF THE WEIGHT OF EACH ⁵/₈" CHAIN

WEEK 1

EXERCISE	WEIGHT	%1RM	SETS/REPS
Bench Press	Chain	TBD	3/7–8
	Free weight	40%	
Bench Press	Free weight	60%	3/12–15
Dumbbell Incline Press	–	–	3/10–12
Dumbbell Flye	–	–	3/10–12

WEEK 2

EXERCISE	WEIGHT	%1RM	SETS/REPS
Bench Press	Chain	TBD	3/6–7
	Free weight	50%	
Bench Press	Free weight	70%	3/10–12
Dumbbell Incline Press	–	–	3/10
Dumbbell Flye	–	–	3/10

WEEK 3

EXERCISE	WEIGHT	%1RM	SETS/REPS
Bench Press	Chain	TBD	3/5–6
	Free weight	55%	
Bench Press	Free weight	75%	3/8–10
Dumbbell Incline Press	–	–	3/8–10
Dumbbell Flye	–	–	3/8–10

WEEK 4

EXERCISE	WEIGHT	%1RM	SETS/REPS
Bench Press	Chain	TBD	3/4–5
	Free weight	60%	
Bench Press	Free weight	80%	3/6–8
Dumbbell Incline Press	–	–	3/8
Dumbbell Flye	–	–	3/8

WEEK 5

EXERCISE	WEIGHT	%1RM	SETS/REPS
Bench Press	Chain	TBD	3/3–4
	Free weight	65%	
Bench Press	Free weight	85%	3/4–6
Dumbbell Incline Press	–	–	3/6–8
Dumbbell Flye	–	–	3/6–8

WEEK 6

EXERCISE	WEIGHT	%1RM	SETS/REPS
Bench Press	Chain	TBD	3/3
	Free weight	70%	
Bench Press	Free weight	90%	3/2–4
Dumbbell Incline Press	–	–	3/4–6
Dumbbell Flye	–	–	3/6

OFF THE CHAIN

USE THESE RECOMMENDED CHAIN WEIGHTS BASED ON YOUR 1RM

1RM BENCH PRESS	SUGGESTED CHAIN WEIGHT	1RM SQUAT	SUGGESTED CHAIN WEIGHT
< 200 pounds	20–30 pounds	< 200 pounds	40–50 pounds
200–400 pounds	40–50 pounds	200–400 pounds	50–60 pounds
400–500 pounds	80–90 pounds	400–500 pounds	60–70 pounds
		500–600 pounds	80–90 pounds

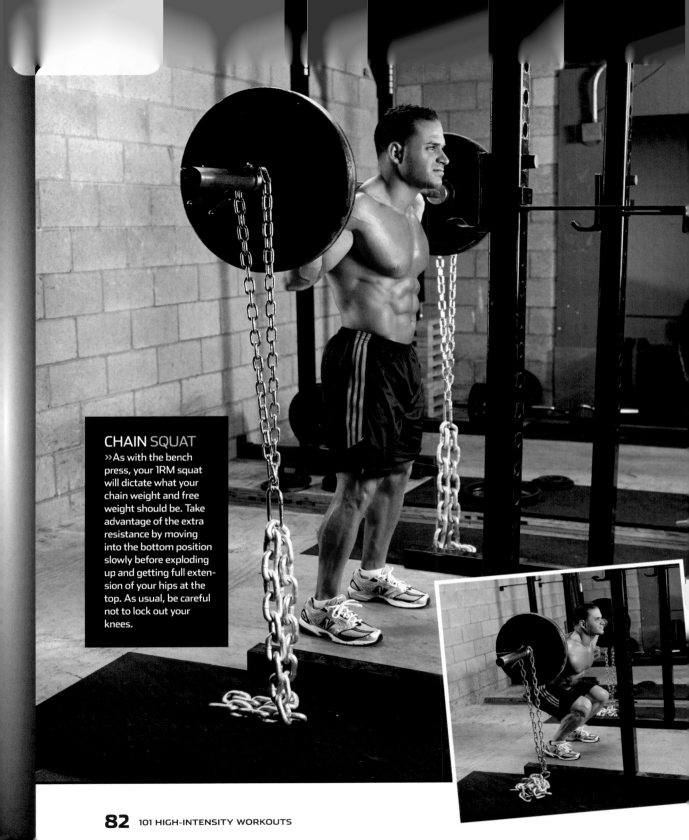

CHAIN SQUAT

»As with the bench press, your 1RM squat will dictate what your chain weight and free weight should be. Take advantage of the extra resistance by moving into the bottom position slowly before exploding up and getting full extension of your hips at the top. As usual, be careful not to lock out your knees.

SQUAT Chain Program

FOR CHAIN WEIGHT, SEE "OFF THE CHAIN" TO DETERMINE HOW MUCH RESISTANCE TO USE.
REMEMBER, $3/8$" CHAINS WEIGH 5 POUNDS EACH; $5/8$" CHAINS WEIGH 20 POUNDS

WEEK 1

EXERCISE	WEIGHT	%1RM	SETS/REPS
Squat	Chain	TBD	3/7–8
	Free weight	40%	
Squat	Free weight	60%	3/12–15
Smith Machine Front Squat	–	–	3/10–12
Leg Extension	–	–	3/10–12
Leg Curl	–	–	3/10–12

WEEK 2

EXERCISE	WEIGHT	%1RM	SETS/REPS
Squat	Chain	TBD	3/6–7
	Free weight	50%	
Squat	Free weight	70%	3/10–12
Smith Machine Front Squat	–	–	3/10
Leg Extension	–	–	3/10
Leg Curl	–	–	3/10–12

WEEK 3

EXERCISE	WEIGHT	%1RM	SETS/REPS
Squat	Chain	TBD	3/5–6
	Free weight	55%	
Squat	Free weight	75%	3/8–10
Smith Machine Front Squat	–	–	3/8–10
Leg Extension	–	–	3/8–10
Leg Curl	–	–	3/8–10

WEEK 4

EXERCISE	WEIGHT	%1RM	SETS/REPS
Squat	Chain	TBD	3/4–5
	Free weight	60%	
Squat	Free weight	80%	3/6–8
Smith Machine Front Squat	–	–	3/8
Leg Extension	–	–	3/8
Leg Curl	–	–	3/8–10

WEEK 5

EXERCISE	WEIGHT	%1RM	SETS/REPS
Squat	Chain	TBD	3/3–4
	Free weight	65%	
Squat	Free weight	85%	3/4–6
Smith Machine Front Squat	–	–	3/6–8
Leg Extension	–	–	3/6–8
Leg Curl	–	–	3/6–8

WEEK 6

EXERCISE	WEIGHT	%1RM	SETS/REPS
Squat	Chain	TBD	3/3
	Free weight	70%	
Squat	Free weight	90%	3/2–4
Smith Machine Front Squat	–	–	3/4–6
Leg Extension	–	–	3/6
Leg Curl	–	–	3/6

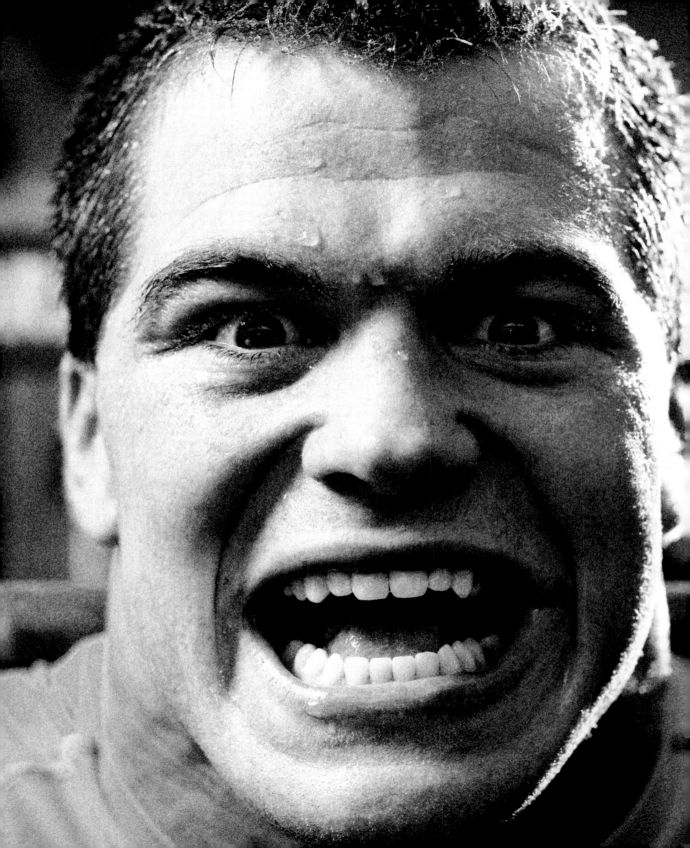

TRAIN
FOR PAIN

THIS FORCED ECCENTRIC WORKOUT GUARANTEES MORE SIZE AND STRENGTH IN THREE WEEKS — IF YOU CAN LAST THAT LONG

Sadomasochism isn't a guiding principle at MUSCLE & FITNESS, it's just a default characteristic that arises from an inescapable weight-room reality: To get bigger and stronger, you have to punish yourself in the gym. Any reader of this magazine has been through that wringer a time or two. We cook up a sadistic master plan based on hypertrophy and pain, and feed it to you with a smile on our faces. It's kind of like serving steak to a hummingbird — if it survives the experience, it's bigger and stronger for it.

So the unapologetic brain trust here opened the big book of pain and ripped out the page on forced eccentrics training. Some of you might be tempted to point out that one man's pain is another's tin-gling sensation, but not this time. The playing field has been leveled for anyone with nerve endings because we're not talking about adding a little time under tension to the negative side of a rep. This is about loading a bar with up to 150% of your one-rep max (1RM) and fighting it all the way down.

To be clear, eccentric training involves empha-sizing the negative or lowering phase of a rep — the unsung and least sexy portion of a move. The concentric, or positive, part of each repetition takes center stage because it requires the most effort; not only are we weaker during this phase but we also have to exert more force than is being exerted against us. Besides, there's a greater sense

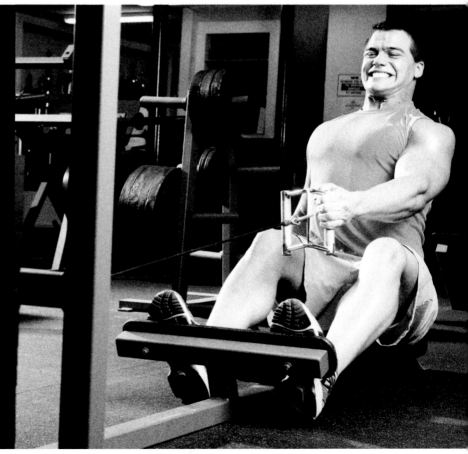

SEATED
CABLE ROW

»Attach a close-grip handle to the cable and sit upright facing the weight stack. Place your feet against the platform with your knees slightly bent. Reach forward to grasp the handle while keeping your back flat and chest up. Drive back with both arms until your torso is erect and your arms are fully flexed, with the handle at your midsection. Keep your elbows in close to your sides as you transfer the load to one arm by taking your other hand off the handle. Keep your torso erect and your head neutral, and squeeze your back muscles as you resist the handle's return. Pull the weight back using both arms, then repeat the negative with the other arm.

SMITH MACHINE BENCH PRESS

>> Lie faceup on the bench and grasp the bar with a shoulder-width overhand grip. Rotate and press the bar up with both arms to unrack it. Transfer the load to one arm, then try to resist the bar as it descends to your lower chest. Press the bar back up to full extension with both arms and repeat the negative with the other arm.

of accomplishment from getting the weight up. Imagine ending each set with the bar marooned across your chest as you wriggle on the bench like an insect pinned to a corkboard. Not sexy.

But there's a method to this painful madness. Research shows that negative training induces the microtrauma to muscle fibers that stimulates the body to repair and build them bigger and stronger than before. (It's also why it coincides with serious delayed-onset muscle soreness.) Part of this stress results in an increase in insulinlike growth factor-1, a prominent ingredient in hypertrophy, and a reduction in myostatin, a negative growth factor. Moreover, eccentric strength is largely used for decelerating and changing direction during sports, so emphasizing this portion of the move in training can help protect against injury.

THE DISCREPANCY

Standard gym equipment is great for concentric overload but can't reciprocate on the negative side without potential lawsuits or unpleasant anatomical breaches. Picture pushing the bar as hard as you can while it descends ominously toward you, unperturbed by your effort. Most true bilateral forced eccentrics are performed with advanced equipment in the lab.

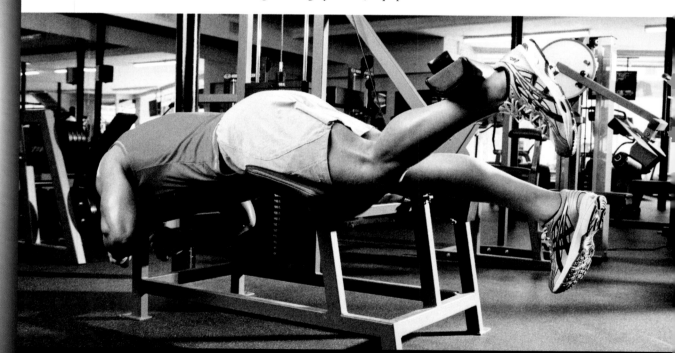

LYING LEG CURL

>> Lie facedown and position your Achilles' tendons under the padded lever; your knees should be just off the edge of the bench. Grasp the handles or sides of the bench for stability and make sure your knees are slightly bent to protect them from overextension. Raise your feet toward your glutes in a strong, deliberate motion. Squeeze at the top, then transfer the load to one leg and try to resist the lever as it descends. Raise the weight back up using both legs, then repeat the negative with the other leg. Alternate sets pointing your toes toward your shins and pointing them back.

THE PROGRAM

This is an advanced and very intense program, which is why you should perform it for no more than three weeks, after which a week layoff is recommended. Do only 2–3 eccentric reps per side per exercise. When you consider that these will be some of the hardest reps you've ever done, and you'll be doing them three times a week, the low volume begins to make sense. Additionally, because forced eccentrics are so damaging, you really don't need many to stimulate growth.

>> **Preparation Phase** The loads used in this program are extreme and will take an unnecessarily traumatic toll on both your muscles and tendons if they're unaccustomed to heavy weights. For this reason, we recommend that you prepare for this program by training with 80% (concentric) 1RM in the few weeks beforehand.

>> **Warm-Up** Since you'll be working with such heavy weight, it's critical that you take time to warm up to ensure optimum safety and performance. Start with five minutes of light cardio, followed by dynamic stretching and two exercise-specific warm-up sets at 30% and 50% 1RM. A subsequent heavy set of four reps at 80% 1RM, using the same movement and machine as in the working sets, will make your eccentrics more effective.

>> **Feeder Sets** Besides pure eccentrics, this workout involves sets with lighter weights and higher reps to stimulate blood flow for maximum nutrient delivery ("feeding") and recovery. Using lighter weight will ensure that you have plenty of energy available during this maximum-intensity three-week program. And trust us, you'll be glad for the reprieve from intensity.

>> **Frequency** Train each bodypart once every seven days.

>> **Weekly Percentage Increase** The percentage of your 1RM (concentric) that you'll use for each exercise will increase by 10% each week. For example:
Week 1: 130% 1RM
Week 2: 140% 1RM
Week 3: 150% 1RM

FORCED ECCENTRICS TRAINING
DAY 1

LEG PRESS	SETS	REPS
Eccentric Sets	2	2 (per leg)
Feeder Sets	3	12–15

Eccentric: Left leg eccentric, bilateral concentric; rest 5–10 seconds. Right leg eccentric, bilateral concentric. Rest 30 seconds and repeat the sequence. These four reps constitute one set. Rest as needed by walking, not standing or sitting, and repeat the four-rep sequence.
Feeder: Do bilateral leg presses using 70% 1RM. Rest one minute between sets.

LYING LEG CURL	SETS	REPS
Eccentric Sets	2	2 (per leg)
Feeder Sets	2	12–15

Eccentric: Start with your toes pointing back. Bilateral concentric, left leg eccentric; rest five seconds. Bilateral concentric, right leg eccentric. Rest 30 seconds and repeat the sequence. These four reps constitute one set. Rest as needed by walking, not standing or sitting, and repeat the four-rep sequence with your toes pointed toward your shins.
Feeder: Do bilateral leg curls using 70% 1RM. Do one set of each toe position. Rest one minute between sets. Cool down with static stretching.

M&F Exercise Science Writer David Barr, CSCS, CISSN, Says: "Only two exercises are used because the leg press recruits a tremendous amount of muscle and induces a high level of physical, neural and hormonal stress. Although the hamstrings are worked in each exercise, knee flexion and hip extension are different enough that there's no superfluous muscle activation."

So, what to do in the gym? Try unilateral machine eccentrics. Single-limb reps are performed because it's neither practical nor safe to perform maximal eccentrics with both limbs simultaneously. The nonworking limb will be used not only as a self-spot but also to concentrically reset the bar for the next rep. A spotter should still be used for optimal safety.

Take the Smith machine bench press, for example. Beginning at the top of the movement, one arm will perform the eccentric portion with a weight heavier than it could press up alone. Once the bar reaches the chest, the other arm is brought in to help execute the concentric portion of the move.

Remember, you'll be using a weight so heavy that it'll be impossible to press it up with one arm, which means the key to getting the best results from this program depends on your effort.

When you start the rep you're not trying to press hard or even very hard against the bar, you're trying to move it with every ounce of strength in your body. If you've only read about intensity, you're now about to experience it firsthand. And you'll appreciate why we have you do only a few eccentrics per set. More important, in three weeks you'll know why the hummingbird eats the meat — if you survive.

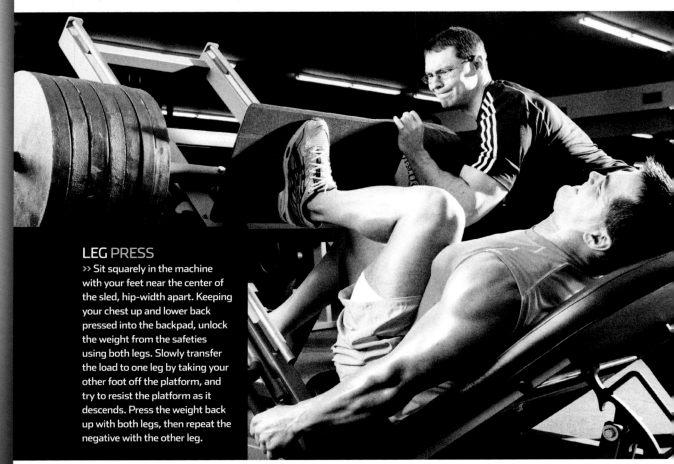

LEG PRESS

>> Sit squarely in the machine with your feet near the center of the sled, hip-width apart. Keeping your chest up and lower back pressed into the backpad, unlock the weight from the safeties using both legs. Slowly transfer the load to one leg by taking your other foot off the platform, and try to resist the platform as it descends. Press the weight back up with both legs, then repeat the negative with the other leg.

DAY 2

SMITH MACHINE BENCH PRESS	SETS	REPS
Eccentric Sets	2	2 (per arm)
Feeder Sets	3	12–15

Eccentric: Left arm eccentric, bilateral concentric; rest 5–10 seconds. Right arm eccentric, bilateral concentric. Rest 30 seconds and repeat the sequence. These four reps constitute one set. Rest as needed by walking, not standing or sitting, and repeat the four-rep sequence.
Feeder: Do bilateral pec-deck flyes using 70% 1RM. Rest one minute between sets.

PUSHDOWN	SETS	REPS
Eccentric Set	1	2 (per arm)
Feeder Sets	3	12–15

Eccentric: Bilateral concentric, left arm eccentric; rest five seconds. Bilateral concentric, right arm eccentric. Rest 30–60 seconds and repeat the sequence.
Feeder: Do bilateral pushdowns with 70% 1RM. Rest one minute between sets.

STANDING CALF RAISE	SETS	REPS
Eccentric Sets	2	2 (per leg)
Feeder Sets	3	12–15

Eccentric: Bilateral concentric, left leg eccentric; rest five seconds. Bilateral concentric, right leg eccentric. Rest 30 seconds and repeat the sequence. These four reps constitute one set. Rest as needed by walking, not standing or sitting, and repeat the four-rep sequence.
Feeder: Do bilateral calf raises using 70% 1RM. Rest one minute between sets. Cool down with static stretching.
Barr Says: "I put calves here because they would be too compromised on leg day."

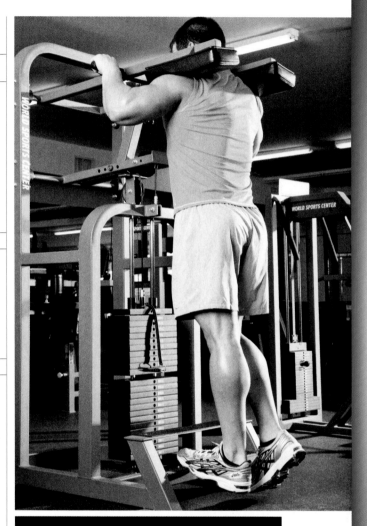

STANDING CALF RAISE

>> Stand in the machine with the balls of your feet on the platform and shoulders under the pads. Press up with both feet to get to the top position. Slowly transfer the load to one leg by removing your other foot from the platform, and try to resist your heel's descent toward the floor. At the bottom, use both feet to press back up onto your toes as high as possible and repeat the negative with the other leg.

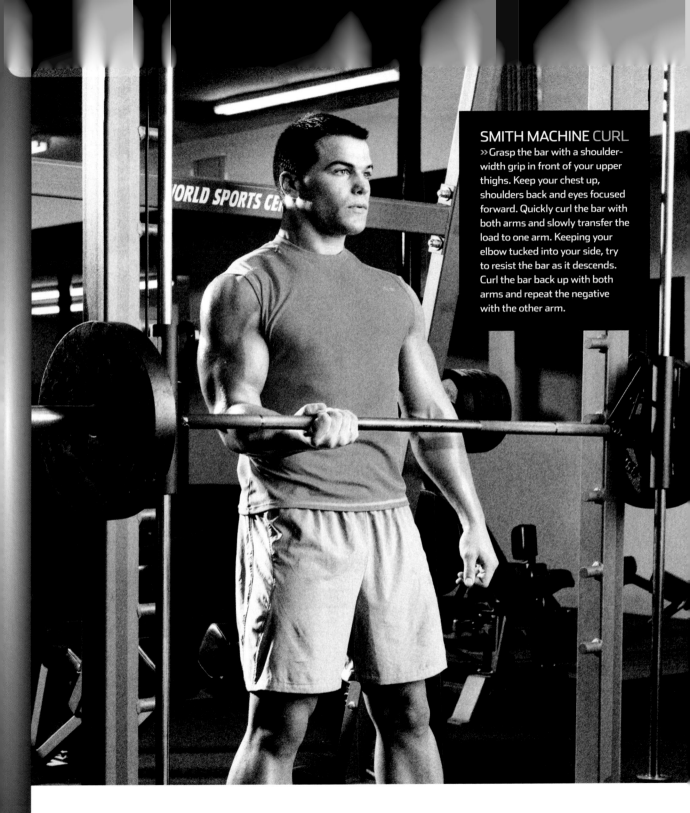

SMITH MACHINE CURL

» Grasp the bar with a shoulder-width grip in front of your upper thighs. Keep your chest up, shoulders back and eyes focused forward. Quickly curl the bar with both arms and slowly transfer the load to one arm. Keeping your elbow tucked into your side, try to resist the bar as it descends. Curl the bar back up with both arms and repeat the negative with the other arm.

DAY 3

SEATED CABLE ROW	SETS	REPS
Eccentric Sets	2	2 (per arm)
Feeder Sets	2	12–15[1]

Eccentric: Bilateral concentric, left arm eccentric; rest 5–10 seconds. Bilateral concentric, right arm eccentric. Rest 30 seconds and repeat the sequence. These four reps constitute one set. Rest as needed by walking and repeat the four-rep sequence.
Feeder: Do bilateral seated rows using 70% 1RM. Rest one minute between sets.

WEIGHTED PULL-UP/ LAT PULLDOWN	SETS	REPS
Eccentric Sets (Weighted Pull-Up)	2	2
Feeder Sets (Lat Pulldown)	2	12–15[1]

Eccentric: Use a stool or plyo box to get into the top concentric position, then perform the eccentric. If you have a partner to add weight, isometrically hold the top concentric while the load is added, then perform the eccentric. Rest 10–15 seconds and repeat. These two reps constitute one set. Rest as needed by walking and do one more set.
Feeder: Do bilateral lat pulldowns using 70% 1RM. Rest one minute between sets.

SMITH MACHINE CURL/ BARBELL CURL	SETS	REPS
Eccentric Sets (Smith Machine Curl)	2	2 (per arm)
Feeder Sets (Barbell Curl)	2	12–15[1]

Eccentric: Bilateral concentric, left arm eccentric; rest 5–10 seconds. Bilateral concentric, right arm eccentric. Rest 30 seconds and repeat the sequence. These four reps constitute one set. Rest as needed by walking and repeat the four-rep sequence.
Feeder: Do barbell curls using 70% 1RM. Rest one minute between sets. Cool down with static stretching.
Barr Says: "Although there are two back exercises, the muscle activation is unique in each. There's a lot of pulling in this session, so if you can't properly contract your back and end up using your arms, skip the biceps curls until next week. Due to the potential fatigue carryover to other exercises, do all pump work at the end of the session."

[1] All feeder sets on Day 3 should be done at the end of the workout.

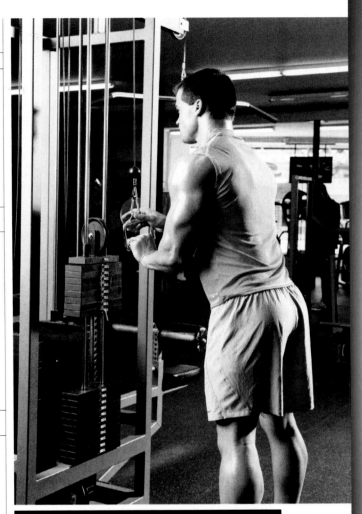

PUSHDOWN

>> Stand erect in front of a high-pulley cable and grasp a D-handle with an overhand grip. Stack your other hand on top to assist with the concentric rep. With your knees slightly bent, lean forward at the waist and pin your elbow to your side. Flex your triceps and press the handle toward the floor until your arm is fully extended. Remove your nonworking hand, then try to resist the handle as it ascends. Switch hand position and repeat with the other arm.

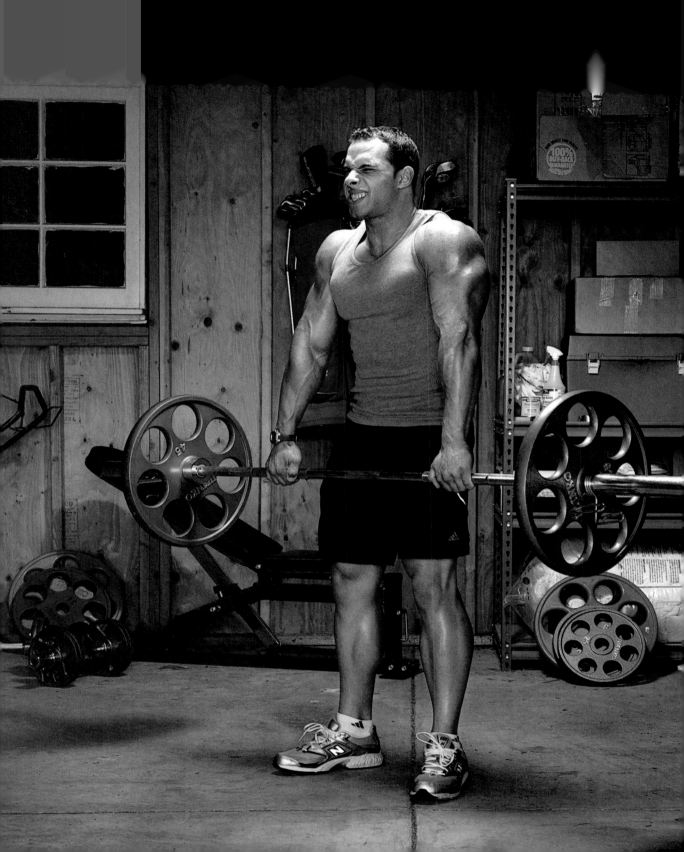

GRIM
REPPER

EXPERIENCE NEW MUSCLE GROWTH AND FAT LOSS — ALONG WITH SOME PAIN — WITH THIS AT-HOME HIGH-REP PROGRAM

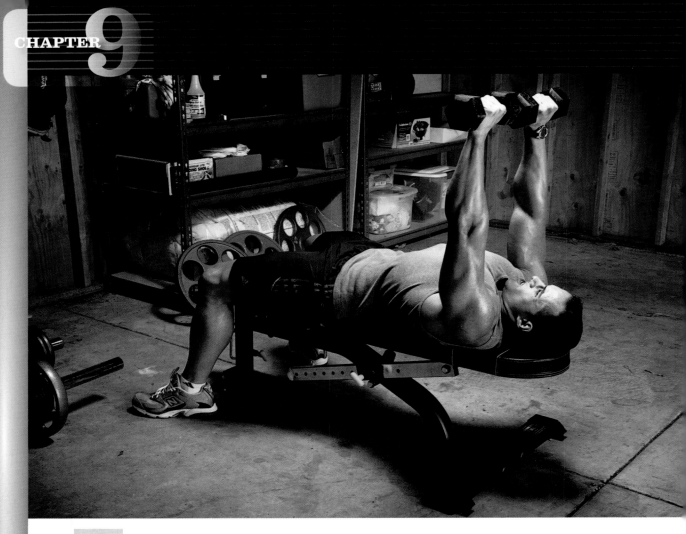

"It changes the person emotionally and mentally." Trainer James "Buddy" Primm is talking about a super-hardcore training method, one he puts his most famous pupil through every Friday for much of the year. That would be Terrell Owens, wide receiver for the Buffalo Bills and owner of one of the NFL's most shredded physiques. Coincidence? We don't think so.

It's called 100s training and, as the name implies, it consists of one set of 100 reps. Each set is so punishing that upon completion it provides the lifter a sense of accomplishment, theoretically making him mentally stronger. "You get [muscle] growth and it burns fat at the same time. It's a total shock to the body," Primm says.

A typical set consists of 8–12 reps, the ideal range for hypertrophy. But sometimes your body needs a little shock therapy to build new muscle and torch bodyfat. Jacking up your reps — even if it means significantly decreasing resistance — can do just that. And it doesn't take fancy equipment or a gym membership. If you own a pair of light dumbbells, a barbell or a set of elastic bands (and sometimes you can use just your bodyweight), the benefits of 100s training are within your reach.

THE CENTURY CLUB

The basis of 100s training is muscle confusion to the nth degree, providing the muscles an experience they've probably never had. The occasional burnout set of 25 reps is one thing, but multiply that by four and it's something else entirely. A set of 100 burns like crazy and tests your pain tolerance,

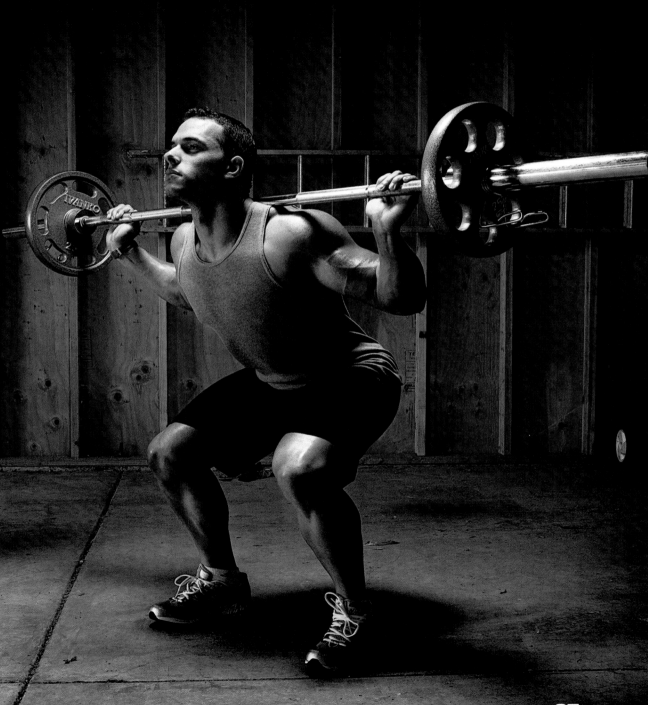

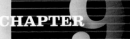

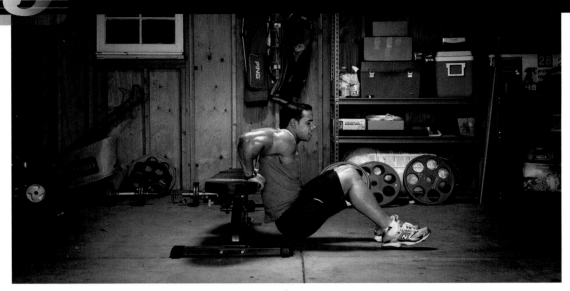

but it's more than just a masochistic display of toughness; the idea is backed by sound physiology.

"[This training] really affects the body as far as taking in oxygen," Primm says. What he means is, such high-rep sets lead to blood vessel growth, so more oxygen plus other nutrients and hormones get to the muscle cells, which in turn increases their growth potential.

Another benefit of 100s is that it effectively trains both fast- and slow-twitch muscle fibers. Because you use a relatively light weight, the endurance-oriented slow-twitch fibers are trained early in the set, when the reps feel easy. As those fibers fatigue

halfway through the set, the fast-twitch fibers, which are responsible for initiating explosive movements, kick in. Most muscles contain 50% slow-twitch and 50% fast-twitch fibers, and by training both in one extended set, fatigue is achieved on all levels.

"On the days I do 100s with my athletes, we don't do anything else. No cardio, no nothing," says Primm, who also trains Tampa Bay Buccaneers safety Jermaine Phillips and Buffalo Bills linebacker Kawika Mitchell. "We come in on Friday and do five sets [of 100s], and that's it."

REPPING FOR GROWTH

The exercises you select for 100-rep sets need to be basic moves (see "100s at Home" for a list of appropriate choices), and you must perform them with very light resistance. This is what makes 100s so conducive to at-home training: It lends itself to exercises such as push-ups, crunches and bodyweight squats, so you don't need to own 80-pound dumbbells or hundreds of pounds in weight plates. Even if you're in solitary confinement on Rikers Island, you have no excuse not to try it.

Despite the name of this program, you're not required to perform 100 consecutive reps; brief rest periods are allowed. If you want to rest only 1–2 times during the set, select a weight that's 20%–30%

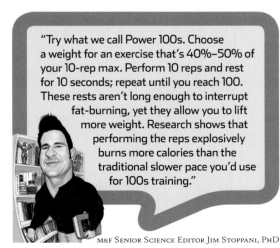

"Try what we call Power 100s. Choose a weight for an exercise that's 40%–50% of your 10-rep max. Perform 10 reps and rest for 10 seconds; repeat until you reach 100. These rests aren't long enough to interrupt fat-burning, yet they allow you to lift more weight. Research shows that performing the reps explosively burns more calories than the traditional slower pace you'd use for 100s training."

M&F SENIOR SCIENCE EDITOR JIM STOPPANI, PhD

THE 100 REPS WAR

Here are two options for 100s training. One involves three weekly workouts of 100-rep sets, which you'll do for no more than four weeks. Opposing muscle groups are paired since training your back, for example, would fatigue your biceps too much. The other is a program to be performed as your last workout of the week, after every bodypart has been trained using low- to moderate-rep ranges.

Three-Days-a-Week Program
Day 1: Monday — Chest, Back, Traps, Abs

EXERCISE	SETS	REPS
CHEST		
Dumbbell Bench Press	1	100
Push-Up	1	100
Flye	1	100
BACK		
Bent-Over Row	1	100
One-Arm Row	1	100 (each arm)
Pullover	1	100
TRAPS		
Dumbbell Shrug	1	100
ABS		
Crunch	1	100

Day 2: Wednesday — Shoulders, Biceps, Calves

EXERCISE	SETS	REPS
SHOULDERS		
Overhead Press	1	100
Lateral Raise	1	100
BICEPS		
Dumbbell Curl	1	100 (each arm)
Incline Curl	1	100 (each arm)
CALVES		
Standing Calf Raise	1	100
Dumbbell Seated Calf Raise	1	100

Day 3: Friday — Legs, Triceps, Abs

EXERCISE	SETS	REPS
QUADS/GLUTES		
Bodyweight Squat	1	100
Dumbbell Lunge	1	100 (total)
Sissy Squat	1	100
HAMSTRINGS		
Exercise-Ball Roll-In	1	100
TRICEPS		
Dumbbell Lying Triceps Extension	1	100
Bench Dip	1	100
ABS		
Reverse Crunch	1	100

Once-a-Week Program
Last training day of the week

EXERCISE	SETS	REPS
CHEST		
Decline Push-Up	1	100
BACK		
One-Arm Row	1	100 (each arm)
SHOULDERS		
Upright Row	1	100
LEGS		
Dumbbell Lunge	1	100 (total)
ABS		
Double Crunch	1	100

NOTE: The exercises in these workouts are suggestions. Use this sample workout or choose from the list of exercises in "100s at Home" according to the equipment you have available.

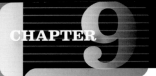

of your 10-rep max. You'll do 70 reps, rest briefly, then continue for 30 more reps.

If you'd prefer to use a slightly heavier weight, pick one with which you can get 20 reps and stop five times before hitting 100. Then, after you've been doing that for a while, you can try doing two sets of 50 and eventually build up to one set of 100. "Kawika had to stop five times on a 100-rep set the first time he did it. It took him about three weeks to build his muscle endurance," Primm says.

As for rest periods, a good rule of thumb is to rest for as many seconds as you have reps remaining. If you need to stop after 50 reps, for example, rest 50 seconds before starting again. If on the same set you reach 75 reps before failing again, you'd rest 25 seconds. Continue until you reach 100.

The key to 100s training is not overdoing it, since sets this intense can lead to overtraining. Primm incorporates 100s in his athletes' workouts only part of the year, once a week and for only five exercises (see the "Once-a-Week Program" for a sample 100s workout similar to Primm's). Another option is to do 100-rep sets exclusively. We recommend doing this for no more than four weeks, then wait at least six weeks before revisiting it.

Either way, 100s isn't for the beginner. "I won't do this with just anybody," Primm says. "It's impractical to do [100s] with someone who's just starting out. You need a good training base. Hundred-rep sets are for someone who's in shape and wants to take his training to another level."

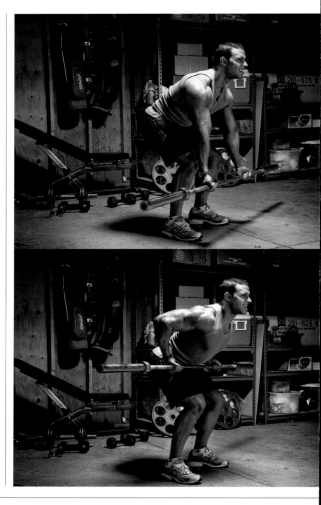

TRAIN LIKE T.O.

This is a gym-based 100s workout that Buddy Primm has been known to put Terrell Owens through during his off-season training. Owens would typically do it on a Friday, after having trained his entire body on a split routine Monday through Thursday.

EXERCISE	SETS	REPS
Medicine-Ball Crunch[1]	1	100
Hammer Strength Incline Press	1	100
Leg Press	1	100
Seated Hammer Curl	1	100 (each arm)
Bodyweight Squat	1	100

[1] Use a 20-pound medicine ball and a sit-up board with a hump, if possible.

100s AT HOME

Don't feel like driving to the gym today? No problem. Hundreds is highly conducive to at-home lifting and requires very little equipment, perfect for a bare-bones setup in a basement or garage. While many trainers say you should use machines rather than free weights on 100s for safety reasons, experienced lifters should be fine with barbells and dumbbells, provided you practice correct form. If you're not comfortable doing a particular exercise for 100 reps (such as barbell squats), pick another move from our extensive exercise list. Then, simply plug the moves into one of the programs on page 99 for a hearty dose of growth-inducing shock treatment.

CHEST
Flat or Incline Bench Press (Barbell, Dumbbells, Elastic Band)
Flat or Incline Flye (Dumbbells, Elastic Band)
Push-Up (Flat, Decline)

BACK
One-Arm Row (Dumbbells, Elastic Band)
Bent-Over Row (Barbell, Dumbbells, Elastic Band)
Seated Row (Elastic Band)
Lat Pulldown (Elastic Band)
Straight-Arm Pulldown (Elastic Band)
Pullover (Barbell, Dumbbells, Elastic Band)

SHOULDERS
Overhead Press (Barbell, Dumbbells, Elastic Band)
Upright Row (Barbell, Dumbbells, Elastic Band)
Lateral Raise (Dumbbells, Elastic Band)
Front Raise (Barbell, Dumbbells, Elastic Band)
Bent-Over Lateral Raise (Dumbbells, Elastic Band)

TRICEPS
Lying Triceps Extension (Barbell, Dumbbells, Elastic Band)
Close-Grip Bench Press (Barbell, Dumbbells, Elastic Band)
Bench Dip (Feet On Floor or Up On A Bench)
Kickback (Dumbbells, Elastic Band)

BICEPS
Curl (Barbell, Dumbbells, Elastic Band)
Incline Curl (Dumbbells, Elastic Band)
Hammer Curl (Dumbbells, Elastic Band)

TRAPS
Shrug (Barbell, Dumbbells, Elastic Band)

QUADS/GLUTES
Squat (Barbell, Dumbbell, Elastic Band, Bodyweight)
Lunge (Barbell, Dumbbells, Bodyweight)
Sissy Squat (Weight Plate, Dumbbell, Bodyweight)

HAMSTRINGS
Exercise-Ball Roll-In

CALVES
Standing Calf Raise (Dumbbell, Bodyweight)
Seated Calf Raise (Barbell, Dumbbells)

ABS
Crunch
Weighted Crunch (Weight Plate, Dumbbell, Medicine Ball)
Reverse Crunch
Double Crunch
Oblique Crunch

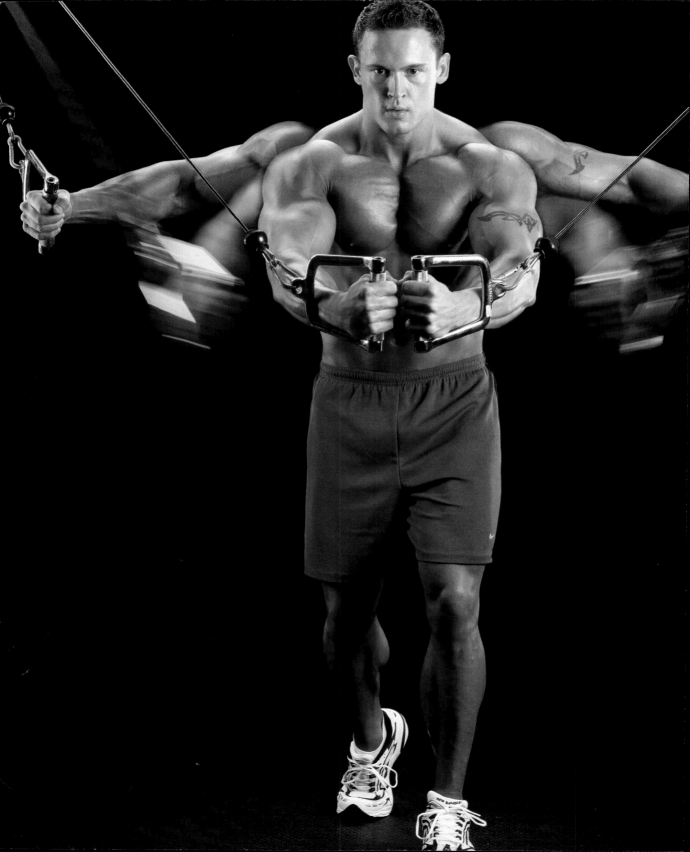

GONE IN THIRTY MINUTES

ON A TIGHT SCHEDULE? MAKE BIG GAINS IN A HALF-HOUR WITH THESE TIME-SAVING **MUSCLE-BUILDING WORKOUTS**

I just don't have time to go to the gym right now. We've heard that excuse from friends, overheard others talking about it, even said it ourselves many times. That means any of our eight 30-minute weight workouts will be right up your alley at some point in, say, the next month.

Contrary to popular belief, you don't need 90 minutes of gym time to build or maintain solid muscle or to get a vein-blasting pump. Some of these routines are full-body workouts while others are for just upper or lower body, but all of them hit the major areas necessary to ensure you train as efficiently as possible when time is short.

A few things to keep in mind: Do each move bilaterally — not unilaterally, or one arm or leg at a time — unless you want to end up doubling your time in the gym. Also, weight selection is tough enough without having to watch the clock. So on our timed workouts, if you end up going too light or too heavy, don't bother repeating a set, which could extend your gym time. Just make a note for your next go-round.

Another good rule of thumb is to perform 1–2 warm-up sets on each bodypart, with certain exceptions, such as when you feel your triceps are sufficiently warmed up after training chest. Same goes for biceps after back and hamstrings after squats or lunging exercises. If doing a few extra warm-up sets means you're in the gym for 32, even 35 minutes, well...that's close enough for us.

Upper-Body Circuit

WHAT: An upper-body routine done in circuit fashion — do one set of an exercise, then immediately move to the next.

WHEN: You're looking for an all-encompassing upper-body blast in a minimal amount of time. Also, when you want to add a cardiovascular element to your lifting, as you take almost no rest between sets.

WHY: Covering all your bases means hitting every muscle group from a variety of angles, which this routine does with three different exercises per bodypart. And because you're training circuit style, there's no need to take full-length rest periods since each muscle group rests while the others are trained.

HOW: Rest between sets only as long as it takes to set up the next exercise. The sequence here is crucial; the exercises can be switched around (or you can pick your favorite moves if they aren't on this list), but be sure to not do consecutive sets or exercises for a single bodypart.

MUSCLE GROUP	EXERCISE	SETS	REPS
Chest	Incline Barbell Press	1	8
Back	Bent-Over Barbell Row	1	8
Shoulders	Arnold Press	1	8
Biceps	Incline Dumbbell Curl	1	8
Triceps	Overhead Dumbbell Extension	1	8
Chest	Bench Press	1	10
Back (traps)	Barbell Shrug	1	10
Shoulders	Dumbbell Front Raise	1	10
Biceps	Barbell Curl	1	10
Triceps	Dip	1	10
Back	Straight-Arm Pulldown	1	15
Chest	Cable Crossover	1	15
Shoulders	Bent-Over Lateral Raise	1	15
Biceps	Preacher Curl	1	15
Triceps	Pushdown	1	15

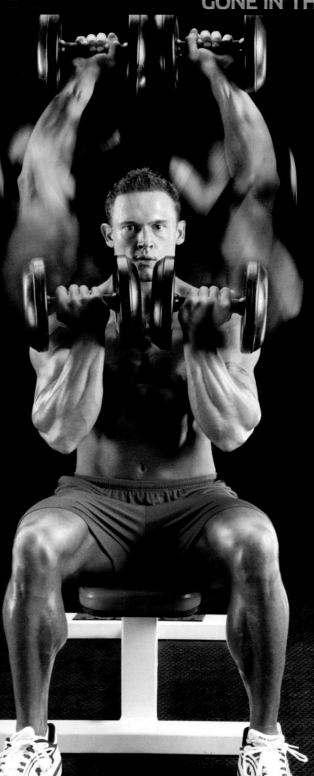

ARNOLD PRESS

» As the name implies, get Oak-like delts with this overhead press.

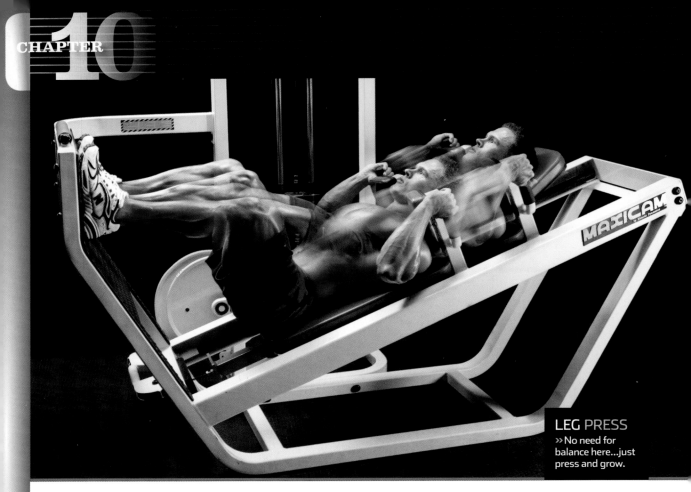

LEG PRESS
» No need for balance here...just press and grow.

Whole-Body Timed

WHAT: A full-body workout that has you doing one exercise per bodypart for time (five minutes) instead of for a particular number of sets and reps — it may remind you of doing rest-pauses. You'll simply do as many reps as you can in five minutes, resting when you need to.

WHEN: You're afraid that doing straight sets will cause you to cut your workout short.

WHY: Some people just aren't able to do 15 straight sets in a half-hour, probably because they're accustomed to resting too long. This "choose-your-adventure" method requires you to train each bodypart in five-minute increments so you never lose track of time. For safety reasons, all the exercises are done on machines — you'll probably fatigue quickly and will be working off of limited rest, and machines tend to be safer.

HOW: For each exercise, select a weight that will cause you to fail at 10 reps. Do 10 reps right off the bat, then rest until you feel ready to go again. Do as many reps as you can, then rest again. Do this for five minutes, which means you'll have to keep a close eye on the clock or your watch.

MUSCLE GROUP	EXERCISE	TIME
Chest	Chest Press Machine	5 minutes
Legs	Leg Press	5 minutes
Shoulders	Lateral Raise Machine	5 minutes
Back	Lat Pulldown or Seated Row	5 minutes
Triceps	Pushdown	5 minutes
Biceps	Machine Preacher Curl	5 minutes

These are sample exercises; feel free to mix in your favorites for each bodypart from week to week.

At-Home Legs + Chest + Abs

WHAT: A routine for the quads, glutes, hams, pecs, calves and abs that you can do at home with no equipment except an exercise ball — and even if you don't have a ball, it would cost you only two sets.

WHEN: You can't get to the gym, you want to work both upper and lower body and you have about 30 minutes before you have to hit the shower for a dinner date.

WHY: Pressing movements for legs and chest are easy to hit at home for a good, quick pump. Polish off your workout with an abs blitz that'll fry your midsection, and you're set for whatever the evening has in store for you.

HOW: Rest 30 seconds between sets, except when going from hamstrings to calves, calves to chest and chest to abs, where no rest is necessary.

MUSCLE GROUP	EXERCISE	SETS	REPS/TIME
Quads	Wall Squat	2	45–60 sec.
	Sissy Squat	2	10
Hams	Exercise-Ball Leg Curl	2	10
Calves	Standing Calf Raise	3	20
Chest	Decline Push-Up	2	12
	Standard Push-Up	2	10
Abs	Crunch	1	20
	Reverse Crunch	1	20

Upper-Body Pre-Exhaust

WHAT: An upper-body-only routine that incorporates a bit of the pre-exhaust principle into back, chest and shoulders, and one set of 100 reps each for triceps and biceps.

WHEN: You can train only two days that week, and you want to hit upper body one day and lower body the other.

WHY: The pre-exhaust technique involves training a muscle first with an isolation exercise before doing a heavier compound move, which lets you use more weight as adjoining bodyparts are called into play. The target muscle group will give out first since it's pre-exhausted, and the 100-rep sets will shock your bi's and tri's in a hurry.

HOW: Make sure you do the back, chest and shoulder exercises in order — the single-joint move before the multijoint one. Feel free to swap the order of bi's, tri's and abs.

MUSCLE GROUP	EXERCISE	SETS	REPS
Chest	Cable Crossover	2	15, 20
	Flat-Bench Dumbbell Press	3	6, 8, 12
Shoulders	Dumbbell Lateral Raise	2	15, 20
	Seated Overhead Dumbbell Press	3	6, 8, 12
Back	Straight-Arm Pulldown	2	15, 20
	Bent-Over Barbell Row	3	6, 8, 12
Triceps	Pushdown	1	100
Biceps	Barbell Curl	1	100
Abs	Hanging Knee Raise	1	20

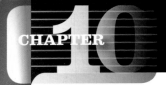

Shoulders + Arms

WHAT: A more focused upper-body workout with no frills — just straight sets and meat-and-potatoes training for shoulders and arms.

WHEN: You're saving chest and back for another day (or you just trained them and they're still fatigued), but still want to get in a quick upper-body pump.

WHY: When time is of the essence, you want to stick to the basic exercises in the 8–12-rep range to maximize hypertrophy (muscle growth).

HOW: Rest no more than one minute between all sets and try to hit failure on each set.

MUSCLE GROUP	EXERCISE	SETS	REPS
Shoulders	Seated Overhead Barbell Press	4	8, 8, 10, 10
Biceps	Barbell Curl	4	8, 8, 10, 10
Triceps	Lying Triceps Extension	4	8, 8, 10, 10
Forearms	Reverse Curl	2	15

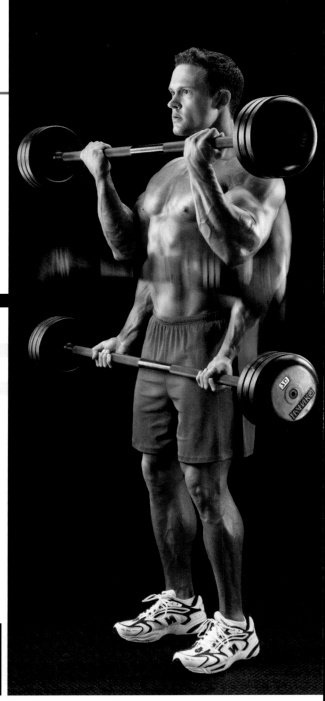

BARBELL CURL
» Arguably the best biceps exercise for great guns.

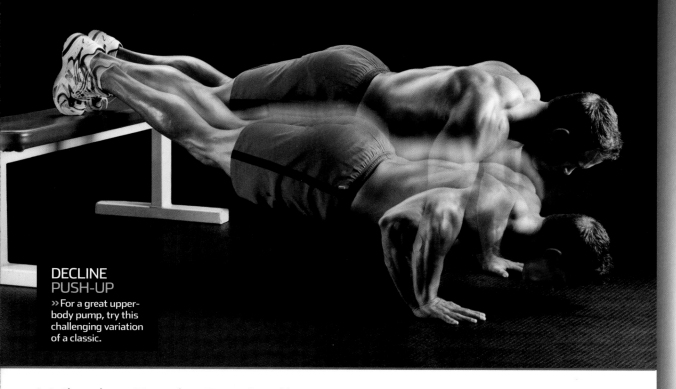

DECLINE PUSH-UP
» For a great upper-body pump, try this challenging variation of a classic.

Whole-Body Barbell Routine

WHAT: A full-body workout that incorporates primarily barbell exercises, the exceptions being the standing calf raise (machine) and crunch (no equipment necessary). Lying triceps extensions can be done with an EZ-bar.

WHEN: You're strapped for time and you don't know if you'll be able to get to the gym the rest of the week.

WHY: With only 30 minutes to hit all your major muscle groups, your best bet is to do compound moves with the heaviest resistance possible — you simply cannot lift as much weight with dumbbells as you can with barbells for most exercises.

HOW: Do not perform this as a circuit. Complete two sets of an exercise before moving to the next. Rest 30 seconds between sets of the same exercise and only as long as it takes to get to the next exercise. For added intensity, after your second set, drop the weight 30% and rep to failure.

MUSCLE GROUP	EXERCISE	SETS	REPS
Legs	Barbell Squat	2	6, 8
Back	Bent-Over Barbell Row	2	6, 8
Chest	Incline Barbell Press	2	6, 8
Shoulders	Seated Barbell Overhead Press	2	6, 8
Triceps	Lying Triceps Extension	2	6, 8
Biceps	Barbell Curl	2	6, 8
Calves	Standing Calf Raise	1	25
Abs	Crunch	1	25

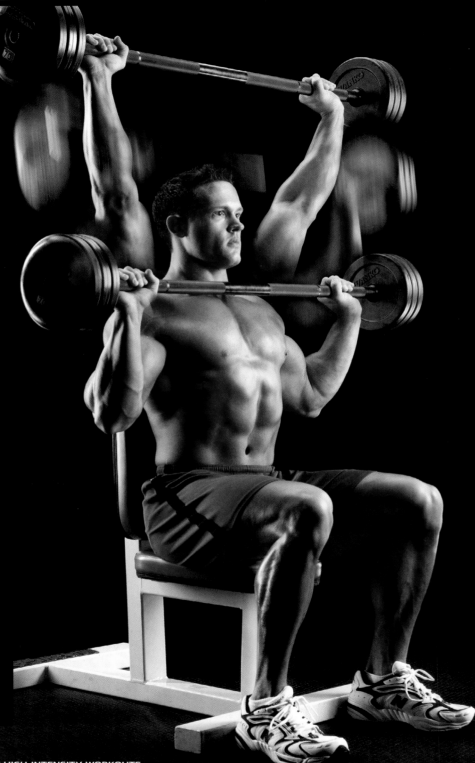

SEATED BARBELL OVERHEAD PRESS

›› Gain overall size and strength with this must-do delt move.

Lower-Body Smith Machine

WHAT: A legs-only routine that requires nothing more than a Smith machine and some plates.

WHEN: You've already trained your upper body this week and this 30-minute window is your only opportunity to hit legs until next week.

WHY: Because chances are you'd have to wait in line at the leg press, leg extension and leg curl machines, or all of the above, and you just don't have time for that today.

HOW: Even though you'll be training fairly heavy with sets of six and eight on squats, limit rest periods to one minute.

MUSCLE GROUP	EXERCISE	SETS	REPS
Quads/glutes, hams	Smith-Machine Squat	4	6, 8, 10, 12
Quads/glutes, hams	Smith-Machine Lunge	3	10, 12, 15
Hamstrings, glutes	Smith-Machine Romanian Deadlift	3	10, 12, 15
Calves	Smith-Machine Calf Raise	4	10, 15, 20, 25

Whole-Body Machine Circuit

WHAT: A full-body routine using nothing but selectorized (Cybex-type) machines.

WHEN: You have only one day to train that week and it needs to hit every bodypart, and you want a hybrid of heavy (sets of five reps) and moderate intensity (12s).

WHY: Using machines means you don't have to rack weights, so you can do more sets in the same time span. Machines let you overload the muscles without needing to balance the weight as with dumbbell and barbell moves, and they give continuous tension throughout the range of motion.

HOW: Circuit fashion, do your first set of each exercise with a heavy weight (five reps), rest one minute, then move to the next exercise. After going through the circuit once using low reps (five), begin the circuit again; this time, lighten the weight and do sets of 12, resting a maximum of 30 seconds between sets. This will provide a great pump and add a cardio element to the last half of the routine.

MUSCLE GROUP	EXERCISE	SETS	REPS
Legs	Leg Press	2	5, 12
	Leg Extension	2	5, 12
	Leg Curl	2	5, 12
Back	Lat Pulldown	2	5, 12
	Machine Row	2	5, 12
Chest	Chest Press	2	5, 12
	Machine Flye	2	5, 12
Shoulders	Shoulder Press	2	5, 12
	Lateral Raise Machine	2	5, 12
Arms	Triceps Press	2	5, 12
	Biceps Curl	2	5, 12

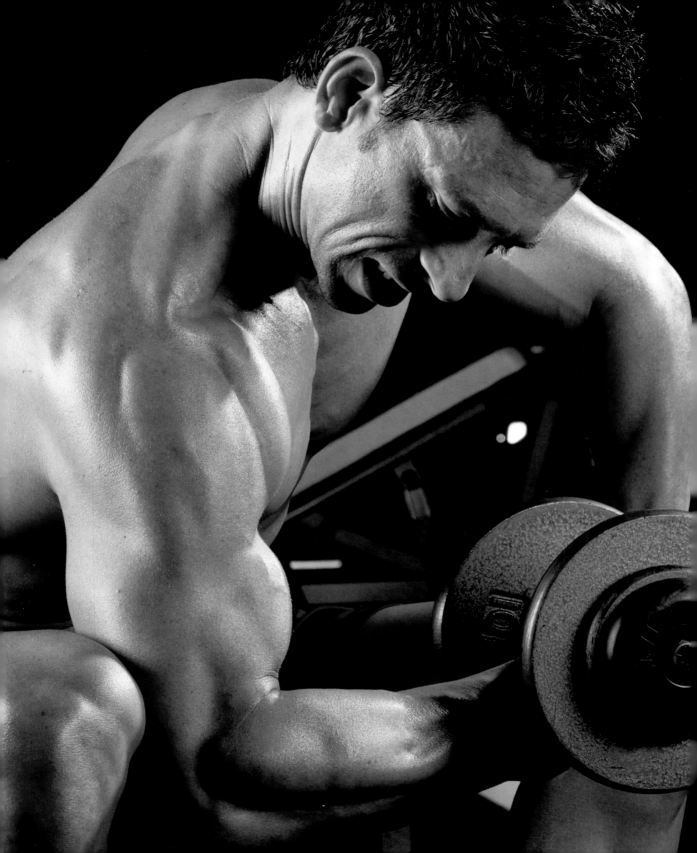

CHAPTER 11

TRAINING
NOTEBOOK

IF YOUR CURRENT ROUTINE IS GETTING STALE, THIS CHAPTER OFFERS BODYPART-SPECIFIC WORKOUTS YOU CAN USE TO INTENSIFY YOUR TRAINING

CHEST
SMALL ANGLES, BIG RESULTS

Make slight bench adjustments on each set to build a bigger chest

While you may be accustomed to thinking that working the chest consists of only three angles (flat, incline and decline bench), the reality is that you'll better develop maximal muscle fibers in the chest if you add even more variety to a given exercise. Hence, doing incline presses from a number of bench angles, and flat benches with a slight incline or decline as well, works the pecs from a number of small angles, each recruiting the muscle fibers a bit differently.

All you need are an adjustable bench that allows for a number of inclined settings and a pair of dumbbells (a lighter set for flyes, though you may have to adjust the weight as you fatigue to reach the target rep) to power through this multi-angle chest workout. You can even apply this small-angle training principle to your barbell moves (for exam-

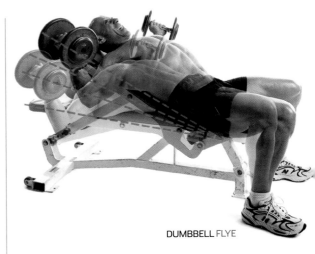

DUMBBELL FLYE

ple, using a normal to very wide grip on your chest-pressing moves) and cable crossovers (lowering the adjustable pulleys from one set to the next) to ensure you're thoroughly hitting all your pec fibers.

Once you see how complete your chest training is with various angles, you'll apply this principle to other bodyparts — if you're not already.

MULTI-ANGLE CHEST WORKOUT

EXERCISE	SETS[1]	REPS[2]
Incline Dumbbell Press (3[3] notches up)	1	10
Incline Dumbbell Press (1[3] notch up)	1	6
Flat-Bench Dumbbell Press	1	6
Incline Dumbbell Press (1[3] notch up)	1	8
Incline Dumbbell Press (3[3] notches up)	1	10
Flat-Bench Dumbbell Flye	1	10
Incline Dumbbell Flye (1[3] notch up)	1	8–10
Incline Dumbbell Flye (3[3] notches up)	1	8–10
Incline Dumbbell Flye (1[3] notch up)	1	10–12
Flat-Bench Dumbbell Flye	1	10–12

[1] Doesn't include warm-up sets. [2] Choose your weights to approach muscle failure by the rep listed. [3] Starting with the flat-bench position, raise the adjustable bench the designated number of stops.

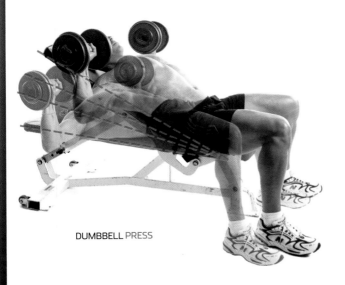

DUMBBELL PRESS

BACK IN THE GAME

Use this routine to turn around your rear view

Is your back playing catch-up with your chest and arms? Then try this back routine on for size. After a few warm-up sets of pull-ups, head over to the power rack, remove the safeties and place a bar inside the rack for deadlifts. Begin with the bar touching your shins. Keeping your arms straight and back flat, drag the bar up your legs until you're standing upright. At the top, squeeze your thighs and glutes hard before lowering the bar back toward the floor.

After deads, insert the safeties into the power rack so that a bar placed across them rests at or just below knee level. From here, perform bent-over rows, but allow the bar to settle on the safeties between each rep before powering it up toward your abs.

Head over to a high bar to perform weighted pull-ups, attaching a dumbbell or weight plate to a belt. Go to failure on each set, and after your last set, drop the weight and continue doing pull-ups until you fail again. Finish up by isolating your lats with the decline pullover, using a lighter weight you can control.

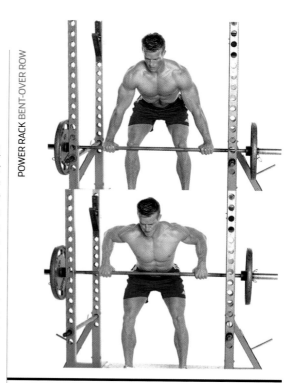

POWER RACK BENT-OVER ROW

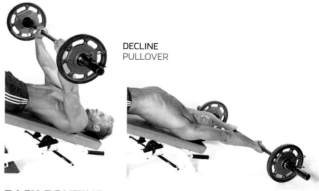

DECLINE PULLOVER

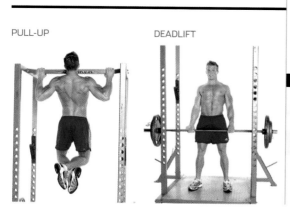

PULL-UP

DEADLIFT

BACK ROUTINE

EXERCISE	SETS	REPS
Pull-Up	2[1]	10–15
Deadlift	2	6,10
Power Rack Bent-Over Row	3	6,10
Weighted Pull-Up	3[2]	to failure
Decline Pullover	2	12–15

[1] Lightweight warm-up sets. [2] On your last set, remove the weight and continue doing pull-ups until you reach failure again.

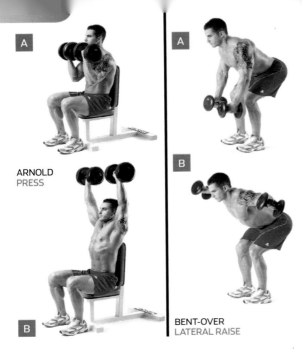

ARNOLD
PRESS

BENT-OVER
LATERAL RAISE

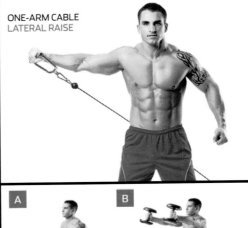

ONE-ARM CABLE
LATERAL RAISE

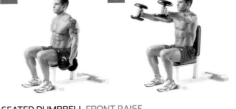

SEATED DUMBBELL FRONT RAISE

SHOULDERS
SHOULDER THE LOAD

Don't let your delts take a back seat. Cap off your V-taper with this well-rounded routine

The greatest thing about training delts is that you'll never run out of exercises. Being a ball-and-socket joint, the shoulder moves across multiple planes and initiates such exercises as front raises, lateral raises, bent-over lateral raises, upright rows and overhead presses. Multiply that by all the lifting equipment available — barbells, dumbbells, cables, plate-loaded machines and more — and the possibilities are plentiful. Yet somehow there are tons of guys whose delts are still unbalanced. Whether it's the front delts overpowering the rear delts or the middle delts hogging all the attention, a change is in order.

With this workout, you won't have to worry about any of your three deltoid heads getting the shaft. You'll start with a standard overhead barbell press to add mass to the middle and front heads. The reps are on the low end of the hypertrophy range (8–12) and rest periods are a bit lengthy (two minutes), so go as heavy as you can while still maintaining proper form. Use a spotter both for safety and to help you get a forced rep or two on your last couple of sets.

After presses you'll move on to a tri-set of raises, one for each delt head. Go right from one exercise to the next, resting only as long as it takes to walk to the next piece of equipment; rest two minutes between each tri-set.

If you can't lift your arms afterward, that's a good thing. Don't worry, your delts will recover.

DELT DEMOLITION

EXERCISE	SETS	REPS	REST
Seated Overhead Barbell Press	3	8	2 min.
TRI-SET:			
Seated Dumbbell Front Raise	3–4	12	2 min.[1]
Cable Lateral Raise	3–4	12	
Bent-Over Lateral Raise	3–4	12	

[1] Between each tri-set

LEGS
THE WHEEL DEAL

It's time to put intensity back into leg day with this brutal blast

No bells. No whistles. You need a no-nonsense leg workout, one that'll destroy your pins and leave your balance wobbly — all in less than an hour. If that describes your current predicament, you've turned to the right page.

You'll start by warming up with leg extensions for a couple of sets, driving a lot of blood around the knee joints. Next, you'll go directly to a heavy weight, about your six-rep max. Hit a set of six, then immediately lighten the weight by a few plates and keep going. When you fail again, drop the weight again. Continue until you've failed a total of four times, including your first set of six.

The key is to make sure you're failing on every drop; don't just stop because you've hit a certain number. A full set may look like this: six reps, then seven, then nine, and finally 12 on the last drop. Do that entire sequence twice.

From there, move to the Smith machine for squats. After squats, turn your attention to hamstrings with Smith romanian deadlifts, again with drop sets. Continue the workout with a leg curl sequence that mirrors the leg extension, starting with two sets of 20, and wrap things up with hack squat calf raises to blast your lower legs.

That's it — 14 sets and you're done. Of course, you won't need to let your legs know that, because they'll be telling you, loud and clear. We'll see you down the road.

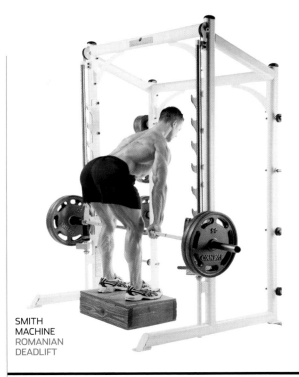

SMITH MACHINE ROMANIAN DEADLIFT

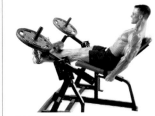

LEG EXTENSION

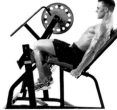

SEATED LEG CURL

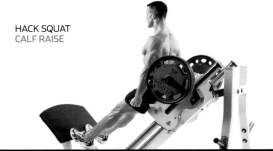

HACK SQUAT CALF RAISE

LEG DAY

EXERCISE	SETS	REPS
Leg Extension	2	20
	1	6[1]
Smith Machine Squat	2	8[1]
Smith Machine Romanian Deadlift	2	8[1]
Lying or Seated Leg Curl	2	20
	1	6[1]
Hack Squat Calf Raise	4	30

[1] Use a weight that causes you to fail at the rep listed. Immediately drop the weight upon failure by 20%–30% and continue until you reach failure again. Repeat once more without rest. Rest at least two minutes, then repeat as indicated.

TRICEPS
TRICEPS TAKEOVER

If less-than-optimal arm size has you looking for bargains on long sleeves, this is one routine you've got to "tri"

Whether you're hitting tri's after chest, coupling them with bi's or giving them a day of their own, this workout is sure to add size and strength to the backs of your arms. The first exercise is actually three moves in one: a lying triceps extension, a triceps pullover and a close-grip bench press. Sound brutal? It is. That's why it's important to be thoroughly warmed up.

Lie faceup on a flat bench and either position the barbell at the end of the bench or have a partner hand you the weight. Take a close, overhand grip and hold the bar above your face, arms extended. Do one full rep of a triceps extension, keeping your upper arms stationary while lowering the bar to the top of your forehead, pausing about an inch from your head and pressing it back up.

Immediately bring the bar toward your head as if to do another extension, yet move your upper arms back to allow the bar to move down past your head. When the bar comes to a point a few inches below your head, pull it up and over your face toward your chest, keeping the bar very close to your face. When the bar reaches your lower chest, powerfully press it straight up, squeezing your tri's hard. The entire sequence is one full rep.

Complete your triceps training by heading to the cable station, where you'll attack each head individually.

TRICEPS WORKOUT

EXERCISE	SETS	REPS
Pushdown [1]	2	10–15
Triceps Barbell 3-in-1	3	10
Incline Cable Lying Triceps Extension	3	15
One-Arm Reverse-Grip Pushdown	3	15

[1] This is simply a warm-up move; don't take these sets to failure.

TRICEPS BARBELL 3-IN-1

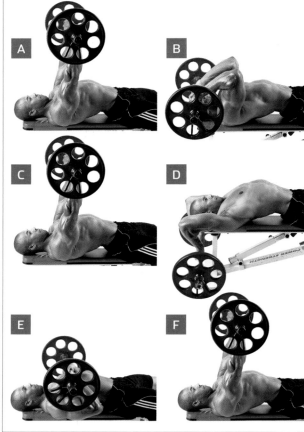

INCLINE CABLE LYING TRICEPS EXTENSION

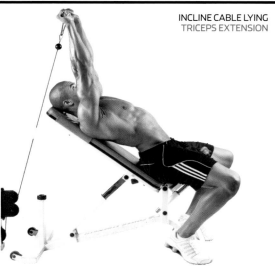

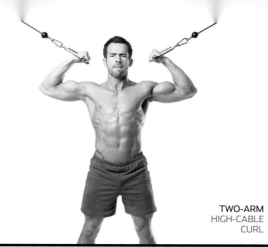

TWO-ARM
HIGH-CABLE
CURL

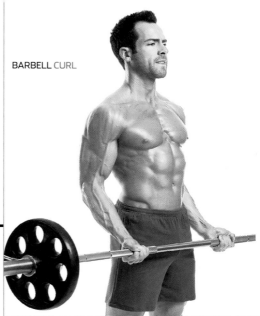

BARBELL CURL

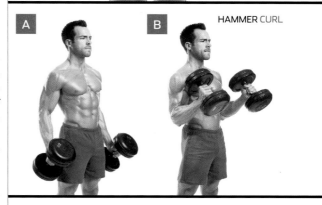

A   B   HAMMER CURL

BICEPS
HAMMER YOUR ARMS

Your biceps called and they sound depressed: They're in a rut and they need your help. You have four weeks

Your bi's are kind of like home-run hitters: They seem to get most of the attention and they're prone to the occasional slump. You hit them hard for a month — maybe even adding a quarter-inch of circumference to your guns — and then the next month they won't budge, no matter what you try.

Designed to get your pipes swinging again, these workouts will attack your biceps from all angles, ensuring that your medial (short) and lateral (long) heads, as well as the brachialis muscle that runs underneath the biceps brachii, are targeted. Barbell and cable curls hit both the long and short heads, high-cable curls target the short head, and hammer curls work both the long head and brachialis. Remember: When a slugger is mired in an 0-for-20 skid, he needs to get back to basics.

These four moves rotate between two weekly workouts to spread the attention between the various upper-arm flexors. Here, on Day 1 you'll do barbell curls first and hammer curls last, and on Day 2 the hammers come before bar curls. Perform the workouts at right for four weeks, then switch up your routine to avoid another slump in arm development.

DAY 1

EXERCISE	SETS	REPS	REST
Barbell Curl (straight bar)	2	12,8	90 sec.
Two-Arm High-Cable Curl	2	12	90 sec.
Hammer Curl	2	12,10	1 min.

DAY 2

EXERCISE	SETS	REPS	REST
Cable Curl (EZ-bar)	2	8,10	90 sec.
Hammer Curl	2	8/8[1]	2 min.
Barbell Curl (straight bar)	2	8	1 min.

[1] Do eight reps to failure, then do one drop set for eight more.

ABS
CRUNCH THE NUMBERS

Carve out your six-pack by adding some weight to your ab exercises

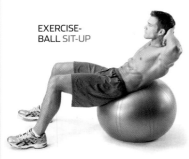

EXERCISE-BALL SIT-UP

If we had a dime for every useless rep of ab work we've seen, well, you know. Most people spend a lot of time trying to get the cubes in the tray to pop out, so to speak, but when it comes to training the midsection, more is not better. Super-high reps won't get those abs to show. While a clean diet and low bodyfat percentage are key factors in abdominal bliss, muscle hypertrophy is the real solution.

Guys get it wrong when they consider the abs to be different from every other muscle group. They train their pecs and biceps to get bigger using rep schemes of 8–12 while doing 50–100 crunches in hopes of chiseling out their six-packs. For some reason, we forget the rules of progression. Rather than doing more reps for abs, try adding weight to your exercises. Every muscle in the human body responds the same way. Increase the training load, which will make the muscle bigger, and those tough-to-see abs will start to become visible.

If you've been doing hundreds of crunches each week in an attempt to whittle your middle, it's time to add some weight to your ab workout. Hit the program at right twice a week with as heavy a resistance as you can handle. Note, however, that the last two exercises aren't weighted. Since your abs will already be tired from the first part of the workout, you shouldn't need additional weight to fail in the 8–10-rep range. Slow down on these exercises to further increase the difficulty. Soon enough, you'll be one of those people who actually trains abs correctly in the gym.

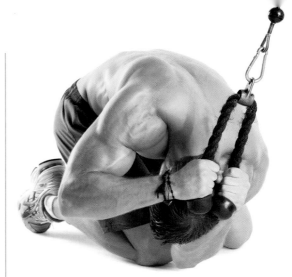

CABLE OBLIQUE CRUNCH

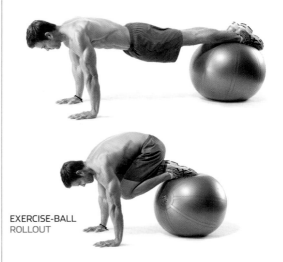

EXERCISE-BALL ROLLOUT

WASHBOARD WORKOUT

EXERCISE	SETS	REPS	REST
Cable Oblique Crunch	3	12 (per side)	90 sec.
Weighted Leg Raise	2	10+drop sets[1]	2 min.
Exercise-Ball Rollout	3	8–10	75 sec.
Exercise-Ball Sit-Up	3	8–10	90 sec.

[1] Do 10 weighted reps, then drop the weight and rep out to failure.

FOREARMS, CALVES, ABS
DETAIL DAY

Complete your training week by dedicating an entire day to forearms, calves and abdominals

Ever been here? Your quads are tired, your chest is sore, and your back and shoulders still need at least a couple of more days of recovery time. Yet you have this dire need to hit the gym. And since this isn't a scheduled rest day, it just seems a shame not to train something.

When was the last time you spent an entire training session on bodyparts that usually get just a few minutes at the end of other workouts? We're talking abs, calves and forearms. It's not that you don't care about these muscles, but you have your priorities, right? Well, today you have permission to rest the majors to hit the minors.

This workout entails a thrashing of these three bodyparts using multiple exercises and varying rep ranges. On some sets you go as heavy as a six-rep max and on others you do 15–20 reps and beyond. As you hit the door to head home, you'll have no doubt that you indeed had something to train.

FOREARMS, CALVES & ABS WORKOUT

EXERCISE	SETS	REPS
Reverse Cable Curl	2	6
	1	10
	1	20
Seated Cable Wrist Curl	3	12
Overhead Hang[1]	3	to failure
Dumbbell One-Leg Calf Raise	3	15
Leg-Press Calf Raise	3	20
Seated Calf Raise	3	20
Decline Cable Crunch	2	15
	2	10
Standing Cable Oblique Crunch	2	20
Double Crunch	2	to failure

[1] Use a wide, overhand grip and hang for as long as possible. Rest as long as you were able to hang on the previous set before beginning the next.

FULL BODY
HIT IT AND QUIT IT

Work your entire body in less time with this all-machine circuit

"I don't have time to go to the gym." Yeah, right. President Obama can sneak in daily workouts, but you're too busy? These days, almost every gym caters to those who have tight schedules but still want a pump. How so? In the form of selectorized machines that are all lined up so you can move quickly between exercises.

This full-body routine was designed specifically for the time-crunched; we estimate it takes 20 minutes to complete. To speed things along even more, do the workout as a circuit with no rest between sets. Perform one set of each exercise, starting with leg presses, and move quickly from one machine to the next. Then start back up at the top and repeat. Notice that the sequence of exercises alternates between opposing muscle groups, and upper- and lower-body moves. This rotation makes rest periods unnecessary, saves you time and keeps your heart rate up for better fat-burning benefits.

The first time through, you'll do a relatively high number of reps to train muscular endurance. The second time through, increase the weight and drop the reps to enhance strength and hypertrophy.

FULL-BODY WORKOUT

EXERCISE	SETS[1]	REPS
Leg Press	2	15–20,8–10
Machine Chest Press	2	12–15,6–8
Machine Row or Lat Pulldown	2	12–15,6–8
Machine Overhead Press	2	12–15,6–8
Leg Extension	2	15–20,8–10
Leg Curl	2	12–15,6–8
Machine Biceps Curl	2	12–15,6–8
Machine Triceps Press	2	12–15,6–8
Machine Crunch	2	20–25,12–15

[1] Perform twice through as a circuit: Do one set of each exercise without resting, then repeat.

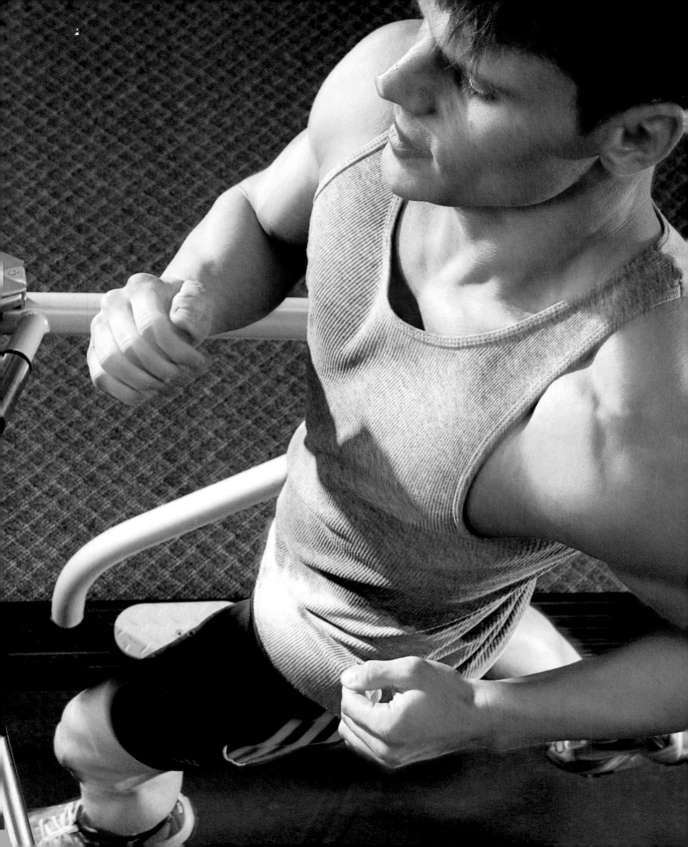

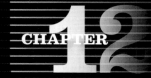
CARDIO FOR THE MASSES

TREADMILLS AND BIKES AREN'T FOR JUST YOUR HEART AND LUNGS. BUILD REAL SIZE AND STRENGTH WITH THESE FOUR CARDIO-INSPIRED WORKOUTS

You don't think Lance Armstrong built his quads in a power rack, do you? His muscular legs were made on a bike. Not that squats or step-ups wouldn't have helped him develop his quads and hams, but the seven-time Tour de France champion is proof that cardio equipment — generally considered to strengthen only the heart — can also build some serious skeletal muscle. Yes, even a treadmill can boost hypertrophy.

"While cardio machines are rarely thought of as a way to increase muscle size and strength, you can actually do both," says David Sandler, MS, CSCS, M&F Advisory Board member and co-founder of StrengthPro and StrengthPro Nutrition, a Las Vegas-based sports-performance and nutrition consulting group. "If you choose very forceful, short-duration, sprintlike activities, you'll inevitably get bigger since there's a direct correlation between muscle size and force capability. Both stride length on a treadmill and pedal strength on a stationary bike require great force, so if you work hard to increase these, your muscles will create more force and increase in size."

The following muscle-building cardio workouts were designed by David Barr, CSCS, CISSN, M&F exercise science writer and author of *The Anabolic Index* (F. Lepine Publishing, 2008). Three of the four routines will help develop leg size and strength, while the rowing intervals will help grow your back, shoulders and biceps. Replace your regular lifting session with one of these workouts every so often or perform it immediately before you hit the weights. Each routine is brief — 20 minutes at most — but far from a walk in the park. After all, Lance Armstrong didn't build his quads by taking leisurely strolls.

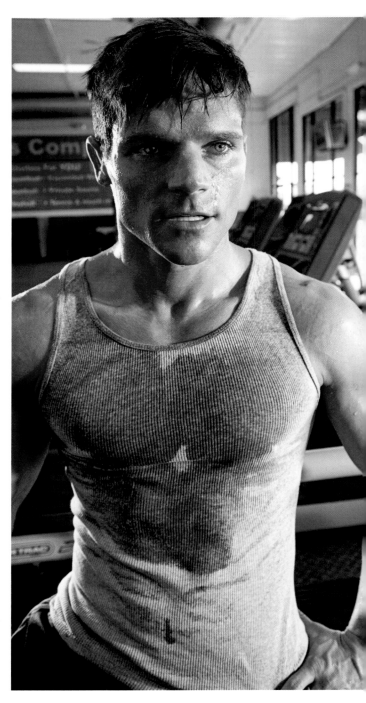

THE WORKOUT: Start with the warm-up and move directly into the first active rest phase. The added challenge of working on an incline makes an 80-second rest period necessary.

WARM-UP: Five minutes of walking 3 mph at 0 incline (heart rate 110–120 bpm)

ACTIVE REST PHASE: 3 mph for 80 seconds at 3 incline (20 degrees) between each working phase (heart rate about 130 bpm)

WORK PHASE: 8 mph for 20 seconds at a 3 incline (heart rate about 160 bpm)

WORK:REST RATIO: 1:4 (20 seconds:80 seconds)

TOTAL SETS AND DURATION: 10 sets (100 seconds each) for a total of 16 minutes and 42 seconds (excluding warm-up and cool-down)

COOL-DOWN: Five minutes at 3 mph at 0 incline (heart rate 110–120 bpm)

ADVANCED OPTION: For 30 seconds before each speed increase, walk backward on the treadmill. The added negative load on your legs is a great stimulus for growth.

COACH'S TIP: "Keep your hands off the handles/railings at all times to get maximum benefit," Barr says. "This may be a tough habit to break, but there's no better time to do it than now."

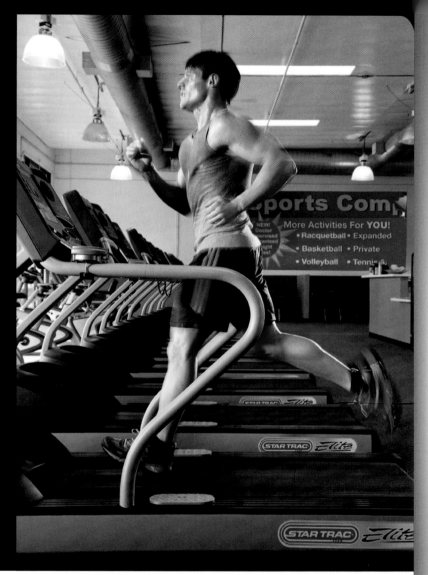

TREADMILL

THE CATALYST: Steep incline, speed

THE REASONING: The treadmill may be most commonly used to torch bodyfat, but it can also build lower-body strength, power and mass if you increase the speed and incline. Granted, you can do uphill sprints outdoors, but finding the appropriate degree of incline can be challenging.

"Sprinting or hard running requires strong and quick ground contact that forces the stride length to be amplified," Sandler says. "Each stride requires push-off strength. Running uphill requires greater force due to the increased demand. Greater force is caused by stronger contractions in the glutes and quads, which means stronger, larger muscles."

ROWER

THE CATALYST: High-intensity intervals

THE REASONING: Unlike the treadmill, stair-stepper and bike, a rowing machine allows you to sufficiently load the back, shoulders and arms for hypertrophy gains. That makes high-intensity rowing a good way to kick off an upper-body session in the weight room when you're looking to bust through a training plateau.

"Pulling harder on a rower means you're creating more force with your lats, biceps, traps and other pulling muscles," Sandler says. "Short, high-intensity bouts on the rower are similar to seated rows. Although it's not as effective at building lat mass as some of the more traditional back exercises such as deadlifts and bent-over rows, it'll still help increase upper-body size."

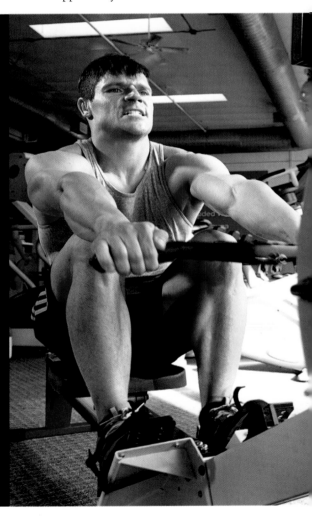

THE WORKOUT: The key to muscle growth isn't the speed of the movement, it's the power you generate during the stroke. Your goal is to pull hard enough that you practically yank the handle off the machine, but then return to the start in a controlled manner. You're not trying to do as many strokes as you can in a given time but rather pull as explosively as possible, even if it means completing fewer reps.

WARM-UP: Five minutes of light rowing (heart rate 110–120 bpm)

ACTIVE REST PHASE: 90 seconds of low- to moderate-pace rowing between each working phase (heart rate about 135 bpm)

WORK PHASE: 15 strokes (25–30 seconds) with maximal effort on the pull followed by a one-second return to the start (heart rate about 160 bpm)

WORK:REST RATIO: 1:3 (30 seconds:90 seconds)

TOTAL SETS AND DURATION: 8 sets (120 seconds each) for 16 total minutes (excluding warm-up and cool-down)

COOL-DOWN: Five minutes of light rowing (heart rate 110–120 bpm)

ADVANCED OPTION: Increase the tension on the machine, decrease the active rest phase to 60 seconds or do more sets.

COACH'S TIP: "Note the similarities between this movement and an Olympic lift," Barr says. "Think *power* at all times."

THE WORKOUT: Alternate between taking one and two steps at a time at a fast pace with active rest (decreasing the speed and doing low- to moderate-pace stepping) between each working phase. Go back and forth from one step to two until you complete 10 total sets.

WARM-UP: Five minutes of light stepping (heart rate 110–120 bpm)

ACTIVE REST PHASE: 60 seconds of low- to moderate-pace stepping between each working phase (heart rate about 135 bpm)

WORK PHASE 1: Fast-paced stepping, one step at a time for 30 seconds (heart rate 160 bpm)

WORK PHASE 2: Fast-paced stepping, two steps at a time for 30 seconds (heart rate 165 bpm)

WORK:REST RATIO: 1:2 (30 seconds: 60 seconds)

TOTAL SETS AND DURATION: 10 sets (90 seconds each) for 15 total minutes (excluding warm-up and cool-down)

COOL-DOWN: Five minutes of light stepping (heart rate 110–120 bpm)

ADVANCED OPTION: Don a weighted vest that's 20% of your bodyweight (for example, a 36-pound vest for a 180-pound individual) while you step. This not only adds variety but also mimics climbing a hill with a backpack.

COACH'S TIP: "Don't forget to drive your knee up as you reach for the next step," Barr says.

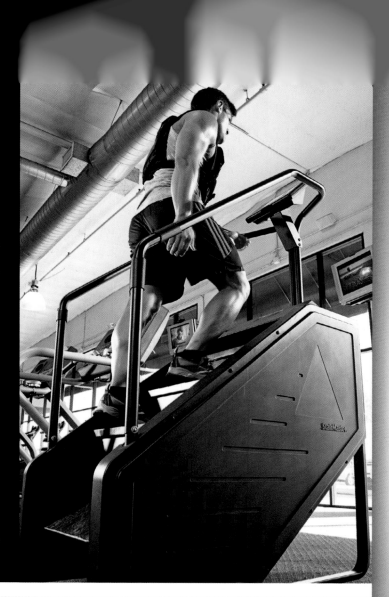

STEPMILL

THE CATALYST: Two at a time

THE REASONING: There are two types of stair-climbing machines: a StepMill, which has steps that revolve around an axis to mimic a real staircase, and a stair-stepper, which has two adjacent pedals that move up and down opposite each other. This workout is designed for a StepMill because it's tougher, Sandler explains.

"You have to actually lift your leg to get to the next step. With a stair-stepper, pressing one pedal down makes the other pedal go up. You'll notice that when people get tired, they lean from side to side, and let momentum and gravity push and lift the pedals rather than making the muscles do all the work."

You can boost intensity by increasing how fast the steps move or skipping 1–2 steps. "This mimics a step-up movement like you'd do with weights," Sandler says. "For additional gains, wear a weight vest for extra resistance to overload your body."

SPINNING BIKE

THE CATALYST: Steep climbs (high-intensity intervals)

THE REASONING: Competitive cyclists are known for having well-developed legs. Lance Armstrong might be skinny up top, but his quads, hamstrings and calves are built, mainly due to his grueling mountain-bike climbs. It seems only natural, then, that you should work Spinning — particularly intervals with high resistance to mimic uphill climbs — into your leg-building program.

"Strength and size increase with greater force application," Sandler says. "While moving a light resistance fast helps build speed and acceleration, it likely won't build up your legs the way heavier resistance will. When strength and mass are the objectives, set the bike's resistance knob so fatigue sets in after 10–15 seconds [30 seconds tops]; make that your working interval. If you can go longer than 30 seconds at a decent speed, the resistance isn't high enough."

THE WORKOUT: The following Spinning routine fluctuates between easy riding (active rest) and very heavy pedaling ("hills"). You'll do a longer session here — 20 minutes total — because your bodyweight is supported, meaning there's minimal muscle damage. This time you're going for continual speed against a very high resistance.

WARM-UP: Five minutes of light cycling (heart rate 110–120 bpm)

ACTIVE REST PHASE: 45 seconds of moderate-pace (70 rpm) cycling at a low to moderate resistance between each working phase (heart rate about 130 bpm)

WORK PHASE: Very high-resistance pedaling (90–100 rpm) for 15 seconds (heart rate about 165 bpm)

WORK:REST RATIO: 1:3 (15 seconds:45 seconds)

TOTAL SETS AND DURATION: 20 sets (60 seconds each) for 20 total minutes (excluding warm-up and cool-down)

COOL-DOWN: Five minutes of light cycling (heart rate 110–120 bpm)

ADVANCED OPTION: Alter the work:rest ratio to 20 seconds:40 seconds by taking five seconds from the rest period and adding it to the hill climb. You may not notice this small change at first, but by the time set No. 15 rolls around, you'll definitely feel it.

COACH'S TIP: "If the longer duration makes you feel as though you're not achieving sufficient speed, stand up for a couple of hill climbs to quicken your pace," Barr says.

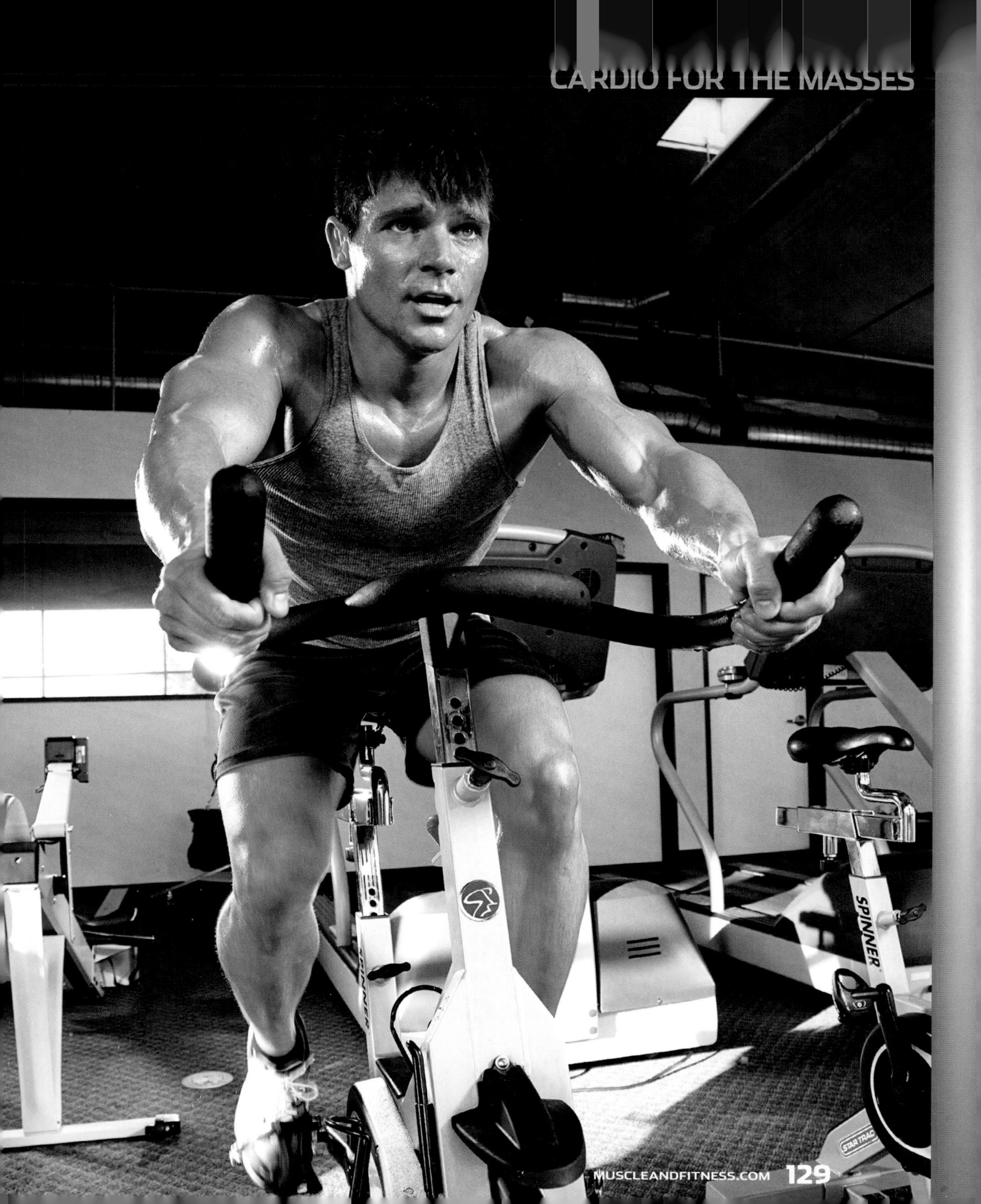
SPINNER
SPINNER
STAR TRAC

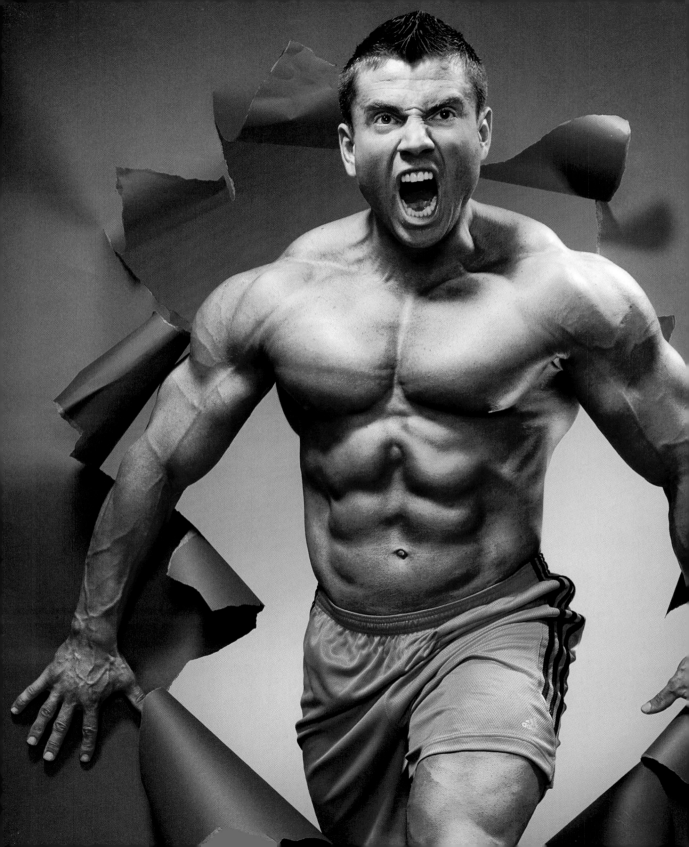

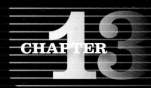
BREAK THROUGH TO A BETTER YOU

IF YOU'RE BEING HELD PRISONER BY A NASTY TRAINING RUT, HERE ARE 101 WAYS TO BUST OUT — AND STAY OUT — FOR GOOD

When it comes to helping you break through your training plateaus, we knew a sprinkling of tips wouldn't cover it. After some discussion, we figured even a "healthy dose" of workout strategies just wasn't enough. A ton? A boatload? Nope — we decided only an avalanche of tips would be sufficient in providing you with the information you need to be your very best. How many tips are in an avalanche, you ask? Well, turns out that after poring over every conceivable way to help you improve your workouts, 101 tips constitutes an avalanche. Now get reading and break through your training rut today!

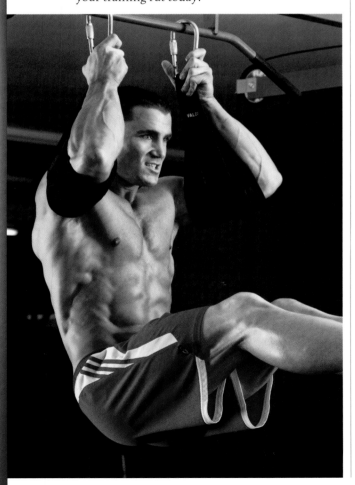

GENERAL

1. KEEP A TRAINING LOG. Only by utilizing a bodybuilding diary can you objectively and accurately assess your progress, isolate trouble spots and devise actual solutions to your problems. Be sure to list every workout — exercises, sets, reps and weight. Include other cogent facts such as personal bests in weight lifted or reps completed, as well as how you felt that day.

2. KEEP TRACK OF YOUR BODYWEIGHT. Check your bodyweight once a week on the same scale and at the same time — ideally, in the morning before you eat — on the same day. During a mass-building program, a realistic weight gain is 1–2 pounds per week. Any more than that and the increase may be in the form of fat. By recording your bodyweight consistently, you'll get an accurate read on whether you're hitting your goals.

3. DON'T ADD TOO MUCH BODYFAT. On the other hand, if the inch you're pinching around your waist is not-so-subtly expanding to 2 or 3, you're overeating. While muscle can grow only so fast, bodyfat can increase rapidly. Keep bodyfat gains to a minimum by eating only slightly more calories than you need to maintain your bodyweight.

4. KNOW YOUR ROUTINE BEFORE YOU WALK INTO THE GYM. Always plan your workout in advance so you're mentally prepared for the training session. Knowing which muscle group (or groups) you'll hit, the exercises you'll use, and the set and rep ranges you'll employ will put you on the fast track to muscle growth.

WORKOUT STRATEGIES

5. FOCUS ON QUALITY, NOT QUANTITY, IN AB TRAINING. You often hear about fit guys performing 1,000 crunches in a session, but you don't hear

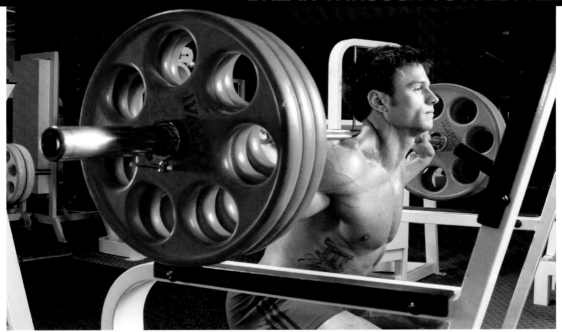

professional bodybuilders say that. Why? One thousand crunches is a cardio workout. It'll burn a lot of calories (fairly inefficiently), but it won't leave behind a ripped sixer. A well-delineated six-pack comes from the intensity of individual ab movements. If you can perform more than 20 reps in any set, you ain't workin' hard enough. Time to add some resistance.

6. **PRESS FOR SIZE.**
For maximum hypertrophy, use the seated barbell shoulder press or Smith machine version. Keep reps in the 6–8 range and do your heavy pressing movements first in your delt workout when you're freshest and strongest.

7. **WORK WITH A TRAINING PARTNER.**
A reliable gym partner provides the necessary motivation to diet and train hard enough to make substantive progress. A knowledgeable, sensitive partner can help make your workouts more effective and rewarding while accelerating your progress. The relationship should be symbiotic, with each of you highlighting the other's strengths and working on one another's weaknesses.

8. **POWERLIFT FOR SIZE.**
Make squats, deadlifts and bench presses the core of your mass-building program. Add other compound movements such as shoulder presses, incline presses, dips, pull-ups, barbell rows, barbell curls and lying triceps extensions and you have a potent routine.

9. **CHANGE YOUR PROGRAM OFTEN.**
Nothing works forever. If you stick with the same routine month after month, your body will adapt to and anticipate that workout, no matter how intense it may be. The end result: Your body will stop growing. Avoid this by modifying your training program every 4–8 weeks.

10. **VARY YOUR EXERCISE ORDER.**
Many bodybuilders start every workout for a particular bodypart with the same exercise. This, however, teaches your muscles to adapt (and subsequently plateau) instead of grow. Change your exercise order every second or third session, adding and substituting exercises liberally so your muscles don't know what to expect. That's what makes them grow.

11. WARM UP APPROPRIATELY.

Start each workout with five minutes of stationary biking or similar cardio option. For each bodypart, perform two light sets of 10–20 reps of an appropriate exercise before starting your working sets.

12. KEEP FOREARM, AB AND CALF WORK AT THE END.

Always do your forearm, ab and calf routines at the end of your workouts. Because you rely on these muscles for most exercises — forearms for grip, abs for core strength and calves for a solid stance — they'll compromise your strength if they're fatigued early in your workout. Always train them after major bodyparts. In other words, keep your priorities in line.

13. TRAIN COMPLEMENTARY BODYPARTS TOGETHER.

To aid recovery, pair complementary bodyparts such as back and biceps — both pulling muscles. With this plan your bi's have longer to recover than if you trained your back and biceps on different days. Another complementary pairing is chest and triceps — both pushing muscles.

14. TRAIN OPPOSING BODYPARTS TOGETHER.

Yes, this is the opposite of No. 13, but if you've been training complementary bodyparts for a while, try pairing opposing bodyparts. This is an equally valid gym philosophy. Train chest and biceps together, and back and tri's. You'll be stronger during arms training.

15. USE TRAINING CYCLES TO ADD MUSCLE MASS.

Maximum strength gains are made possible by dividing your workout year into distinct training cycles. Commonly referred to as *periodization*, this system is based on the fact that continual heavy-duty training doesn't lead to optimal progress. The body instead responds to gradual increases and decreases in intensity, so switch between light weights/high reps and heavy weights/low reps.

16. WORK ON YOUR WEAKNESSES.

Many bodybuilders make the mistake of focusing on what they perceive as their strengths while ignoring their weaknesses. The best athletes concentrate on bringing up their weak areas to achieve symmetry and balance. If a smaller bodypart is weak, emphasize it by training it first after two days of rest.

17. DON'T NEGLECT MINOR BODYPARTS.

With all the emphasis on legs, chest and back, many trainees ignore the smaller muscle groups that complete the picture of perfect symmetry. Be sure to train traps, calves and forearms in your weekly split. If these smaller muscles are ignored, they could end up being weak links.

18. WORK STABILIZER MUSCLES.

A good many bodybuilders develop shoulder, low-back or knee problems because they build their strength and major muscle groups beyond the point at which stabilizer muscles can work effectively. Keep your stabilizers in mind as you train. To avoid injury, add movements such as rotator cuff exercises, back extensions and core moves to your program.

19. USE PROPER FORM.

To develop precise technique, do every rep with good form. Beginners, strive to keep the rep target inside your strength capabilities. Find the right groove for each exercise. Don't train to failure when you're just starting out.

20. CULTIVATE THE MIND-MUSCLE CONNECTION.

Research confirms that tuning in to the mind-muscle connection can optimize your results in the gym. Visualize your target muscle contracting and growing as you complete every rep of every set. Remember, it's not the sheer amount of weight on the bar that's important; it's the effect of that weight on the muscle that leads to increases in the size, strength and power you're after.

IN THE GYM

21. START BASIC. Most workouts for your major bodyparts should start with basic, multijoint exercises that allow you to lift more weight, such as the bench press for chest, overhead press for delts, barbell row for back and squat for legs. This will allow you to lift heavier on these exercises while you're fresh and better stimulate muscle growth.

22. STRAP IT. Research shows that wrist straps help bodybuilders complete more sets on pulling exercises, such as most back moves. To get your back to grow, you need to complete as many reps as possible with a given weight. Worried about your grip strength? Train your grip after the back workout.

23. USE A BELT. A weight belt is a must when you go heavy on exercises such as squats, deadlifts, shoulder presses and barbell rows.

24. BE IN TUNE. Listening to your favorite music while you train can make a world of difference in your strength, research confirms. Use a portable MP3 player with headphones and make sure your playlist is stocked with plenty of music that gets you pumped up for your workout.

25. STRETCH AFTER TRAINING. Research data show that static stretching before workouts not only fails to reduce your chance of injury but can also decrease your strength. We recommend static stretching after the workout as a cool-down when your muscles are more flexible.

26. REST LESS BETWEEN SETS. Taking a shorter rest period between sets can increase the metabolic effect of weight

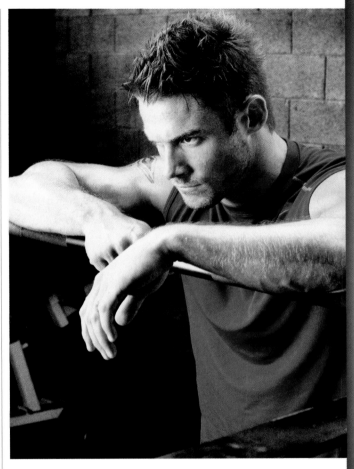

training. It also increases the intensity, forcing your muscles to work before they're fully recovered from the previous set. Research also shows that resting less can further boost growth hormone (GH) levels.

27. REST MORE BETWEEN SETS. An opposing but equally effective strategy is to rest longer between sets. Take five minutes between sets of squats to allow for full recovery so you can perform more reps. Learn to use the length of your rest period — whether you go longer or shorter — to intensify your workouts and enhance gains.

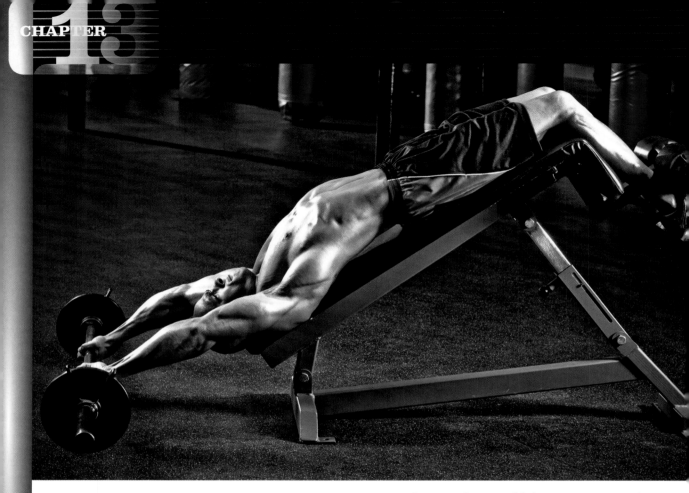

28. TAKE A DIFFERENT ANGLE.

Changing up the angles you use while training will help you hit different muscle fibers in each major group. For example, do dumbbell presses at zero, 20, 30 and 45 degrees. This applies to your grip as well as the bench angle. For example, try barbell curls with a variety of hand-grip widths from as wide to as narrow as you can go. These small adjustments can make a big impact on your muscle gains.

WEIDER TRAINING PRINCIPLES

29. UTILIZE FORCED REPS.

Forced reps are a way to extend a set and maintain intensity beyond failure. When you reach initial failure in a set, have your training partner give you just the right amount of assistance to help you through 2–3 more reps. By prolonging the set past the normal point of failure, you optimize the stress placed on the muscle fibers and therefore overload the targeted muscles. Attempt forced reps during only your last set of a particular exercise. Research confirms that forced reps lead to greater GH levels and enhance fat loss.

30. OVERLOAD THE MUSCLE TO STIMULATE GROWTH.

The key to hypertrophy is forcing the muscle to respond to an increased workload. Using the overload principle continually forces muscles to respond and adapt to a task they aren't accustomed to, so they must adjust by getting strong enough to handle the load.

31. PRE-EXHAUST THE MUSCLE WHEN WORKING LARGE BODYPARTS.

When training thighs, for example, do three sets of leg extensions to fatigue the quads before moving on to leg presses, and use a lighter weight than usual here. These lighter presses help fatigue the quads to the max without putting your joints, tendons and ligaments under too much pressure.

32. TRY SPLIT ROUTINES TO MAXIMIZE EFFICIENCY.
With split routines you'll likely hit a few bodyparts on one day, a few others on another day and still others on a third day. This allows you to train on successive days, as some bodyparts rest while you train others.

33. EXPERIMENT WITH THE REST-PAUSE METHOD.
As with forced reps, you can use this strength-building principle at the end of a set to extend it beyond failure. With machine presses, for instance, rest 10–15 seconds at the end of a set to regain strength, do more reps before another 10–15-second rest interval, then perform even more reps as a coup de grâce.

34. USE PARTIAL REPS TO UP THE INTENSITY ANTE.
When forced reps aren't practical for boosting intensity, give partial reps a try. After reaching failure on an exercise, continue to lift the weight as high as possible — whether that means doing three-quarter reps, half reps or quarter reps — to thoroughly fry the muscle.

35. USE NEGATIVE REPS.
Another way to extend a set beyond failure is to resist the weight as it moves through the negative (eccentric) part of the rep. Lower the weight as slowly as possible to maximize the stress on the muscle fibers by controlling the negative.

36. USE DROP SETS TO MAINTAIN INTENSITY.
Drop sets are practical for anyone training alone and applicable to exercises that make forced reps inefficient or all but impossible. During seated dumbbell curls, for instance, drop the weights at the point of failure and pick up dumbbells that are 20%–30% lighter to squeeze out more reps. Maintaining intensity past the point of failure is the name of the game.

37. USE CABLE MOVEMENTS FOR CONSTANT TENSION.
When you use dumbbells, a feeling of extreme muscular tension doesn't occur until nearly halfway through the upward swing on, say, a lateral raise. With cables, however, severe muscular tension is constant throughout the movement. Add cable exercises to all upper-body workouts to apply continuous tension to these muscle groups.

38. LEARN HOW TO CHEAT.
Use the cheating principle only when you reach failure at the end of a set. When you're unable to complete a full rep with perfect form on, say, barbell curls, bend slightly forward and then backward as you begin the curl, enlisting upper-body momentum to power the rep. This prolongs the set and increases muscular stress. Perform cheating reps on only the last set of an exercise, and then for only 2–3 reps.

39. SUPERSET.
There are few better ways to boost training intensity and reduce gym time than with the superset — doing two exercises back-to-back without rest. You can train one muscle group or two different bodyparts this way. The lack of rest between sets will boost training intensity and GH levels for better growth, and you'll be out of the gym in less time.

40. GIANT SETS FOR A GIANT PUMP.
A giant set is a series of 4–6 exercises for one bodypart done in quick succession. With chest, for example, you could do a giant set of incline presses, pullovers, flyes and dips with only as much rest between sets as it takes to get to the next exercise. This flushes blood to the muscles being worked and greatly increases training intensity and effect.

RECUPERATION FACTORS

41. SCHEDULE REST DAYS.
If your workouts constitute 100% effort — an absolute must for making steady progress — then you need to schedule days off from strength training to ensure adequate recuperation. Spend too much time in the gym and you won't grow! Unless you're preparing for a contest, make a four- or five-days-a-week training regimen your limit. Any more than that is overkill.

42. AVOID OVERTRAINING.
Don't be stubborn about ignoring the signs of overtraining or your workouts will become counterproductive. Telltale symptoms of overtraining include loss of appetite, joint aches, nausea, a negative attitude, trouble sleeping, irritability, fatigue and even a general listless feeling. The cure is to take a vacation from the gym for 1–2 weeks, let your body regroup and then come back like a lion.

43. LISTEN TO YOUR BODY.
Often, bodybuilders go to the gym with a routine already in mind. They're so focused on performing that workout that they don't listen to feedback from their bodies. But strength and muscle gains are made in a cyclical fashion rather than a linear one. Some days you may not be as strong as on other days. Learn to accept that instead of trying to force your body to achieve what's not possible. You can't improve on your previous workout every time you train.

44. DON'T TRAIN UNLESS YOU'RE FULLY RECOVERED.
Too many bodybuilders go to the gym to work out simply because they're supposed to do it that day. While it's important to have a schedule, you should adhere to it intelligently. If you're still tight and sore from the previous week's training or you feel halfhearted, don't force yourself to endure a workout if you think another day's rest might improve your performance.

45. GET A GOOD NIGHT'S SLEEP.
Bodybuilders need more rest than the average Joe. Exercise and weight training place great demands on the body, and sleep helps the body recover better than any other activity. Make sure you get at least eight hours of sleep a night, and strive to get an extra half-hour or so on days you train.

46. TAKE AN AFTERNOON NAP.
When possible, aid your recovery by taking a nap in the afternoon. While it may be impractical for many people because of work or school obligations, take the opportunity when it presents itself to get a little sleep during the day. Even 20 minutes can have an amazing restorative and recuperative effect on the body.

47. INCORPORATE RELAXATION TECHNIQUES.
Relaxation leads to recovery. It helps reduce levels of the catabolic hormone cortisol, which competes with testosterone, so relaxing can indirectly help you boost your T levels. Relaxation techniques can be as simple as spending an evening watching TV, listening to calming music or getting a massage. Yoga, stretching, acupuncture, acupressure and hydrotherapy can also be effective.

48. TAKE A WEEK OFF.
The body needs an occasional respite from the gym. Taking a one-week break every 3–4 months allows you to mentally and physically recover from the rigors of balls-out training. Plus, your muscles grow during recovery, not during workouts, and a one-week period of active rest can be beneficial to achieving your goals.

GENERAL NUTRITION

49. MAINTAIN CONSISTENCY.
Bodybuilding workouts are best done an average of 4–5 times per week. Bodybuilding nutrition is best done an average of seven days

a week, every week. While you'll make adjustments from day to day depending on your goals, you must be consistent with your diet.

50. **EAT FOR SIZE.**
Many bodybuilders are hardgainers, and they learned to overcome this genetic predisposition by eating for size. Eating a few extra quality calories at every meal adds up over the course of the day. The bodybuilder who eats just past satisfaction is the one who will consume the extra calories necessary for growth.

51. **EAT SEVERAL MEALS A DAY.**
One of the most challenging aspects of being a bodybuilder is eating the requisite meals. Trainees often have huge appetites because of their caloric expenditure, and they're able to consume large quantities in one sitting. To most effectively get what you need from your calories, however, a better strategy is to divide your intake over six — if not 7–8 — snacks/meals each day.

52. **EAT BALANCED MEALS.**
If you think bodybuilding nutrition is all about protein, think again. It's really about providing your body with the optimal balance of foods at every meal. Eat a balance of protein, slow-digesting carbs, healthy fats and vegetables.

53. **KEEP NUTRIENT INTAKE STEADY THROUGHOUT THE DAY.**
Part of the reason behind eating several meals a day is to provide your body with a steady stream of nutrients. It's important to not only eat six meals a day but to eat healthy fats, quality protein and complex carbs at every meal to continually supply your body with what it needs to grow.

54. **CONSUME ADEQUATE PROTEIN.**
Bodybuilders know they must eat quality protein — nothing is more crucial to muscle-building. Without protein, you simply can't provide your body with the most rudimentary tool

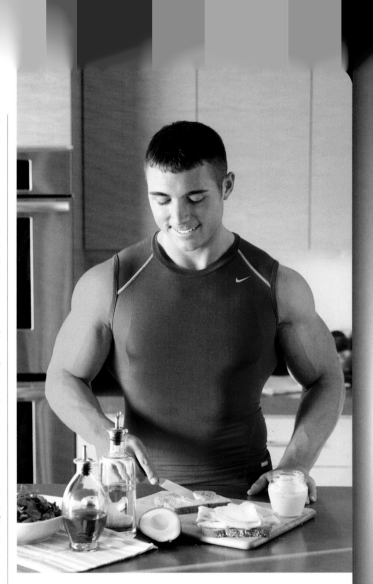

for growth. Make sure to consume at least 1 gram of protein per pound of bodyweight every day.

55. **EAT SLOW-DIGESTING CARBS.**
Gym rats often avoid carbohydrates for fear they'll add too much bodyfat. Most amateur bodybuilders eat plenty of carbs, but they choose simple or starchy carbs at the expense of the more beneficial slow-digesting carbohydrates. Emphasize foods such as sweet potatoes, oatmeal, fruit, brown rice, whole-grain breads and pastas, and quinoa in your diet. These foods, along with protein, most encourage muscle growth.

56. **EAT FAST-DIGESTING CARBS.** Okay, we know this contradicts the previous rule, but there *is* a time for fast carbs: immediately after workouts when they'll boost insulin and help drive muscle recovery and growth. Go with 40–100 grams of fast-digesting carbs from sources such as sports drinks, white bread, and fat-free candy like jellybeans.

57. **EAT HEALTHY FATS.** As a bodybuilder, you need healthy fats for optimal hormone production and immune function and for a sense of well-being. Include moderate portions of healthy fats with most of your meals. Excellent sources include canola and olive oils, nuts and seeds, avocados and fatty fish such as salmon.

58. **GET A VARIETY OF PROTEIN SOURCES.** Individual variance prevents prescribing *the* absolute best bodybuilding nutrition regimen. Some lifters swear by red meat, saying they feel stronger when they eat it, perhaps because of the iron and creatine it contains. Others prefer fish or chicken, saying they have trouble digesting red meat. Your best bet is to utilize a variety of protein sources such as beef, poultry, fish, eggs and dairy to reap the benefits of each.

59. **AVOID LOW-FAT DIETS.** One of the worst trends in bodybuilding nutrition was the low-fat diet. Good fats offer many benefits to the body; even saturated fats provide a sense of satiety and fulfillment, not to mention they boost testosterone levels. Without fats, you aren't giving your body what it craves and what it needs to build muscle. Emphasize good fats, but don't completely exclude bad fats.

60. **AVOID TRANS FATS.** There's one type of fat you *do* want to avoid at any cost: trans fats. These manmade fats can be listed on labels as hydrogenated oil or partially hardened vegetable oil. Trans fats not only harm your health but can impair muscle recovery and increase muscle breakdown.

61. **EAT PLENTY OF FIBER.** As a rule, bodybuilding foods don't contain as much fiber as bodybuilders need. The best solution is to eat whole foods that are high in fiber such as vegetables, fruits, legumes, nuts and seeds. Using a fiber supplement is also an option. While these products lack the nutrients of whole food, they do provide the fiber your body needs.

62. **DRINK ENOUGH WATER.** Water is the great purifier, and bodybuilders especially need purification. It's also essential for keeping muscles full, and a drop in body water that's just 2% of your bodyweight can significantly decrease your strength. In effect, the larger you are and the more food you consume, the more water you need on a daily basis. A 200-pound bodybuilder should drink at least 1 gallon of water per day in addition to other beverages.

63. **BREAK THE FAST.** If you're one of those guys who can't stomach the thought of food until a couple of hours after waking up, you'd better adapt. The nightlong fast causes your body to break down your muscle fibers for fuel, so you need to eat protein and carbs ASAP upon waking. Your best bet is a fast-digesting protein like whey along with a piece of fruit.

64. **PREPARE FOR YOUR WORKOUT** Before every training session, fuel up with about 20 grams of whey protein and some slow-digesting carbs. Both will provide long-lasting energy throughout your workout without blunting fat-burning.

65. **EAT IMMEDIATELY AFTER WORKOUTS.** As soon as your workout is over, it's time to refuel with about 40 grams of whey protein and 40–80 grams of fast-digesting carbs.

These work together to enhance recovery and push muscle growth forward.

66. EAT FOR CONDITION.

Calories are essential for growth, but certain calories will more likely spur hypertrophy while others encourage fat gain. Avoid excess sugar and starchy carbs, as these will undermine your condition. By monitoring your diet, you can maintain conditioning and add muscle.

67. AVOID FEELING HUNGRY.

When you're hungry, you're in a potentially catabolic state in which your body uses muscle tissue for energy. Once your blood sugar dips below a certain level, your body begins to search for another source of energy, and it turns to muscle much more readily than bodyfat. Take that sense of hunger as a warning that your muscles are under siege, and fight it off with a well-balanced bodybuilding meal.

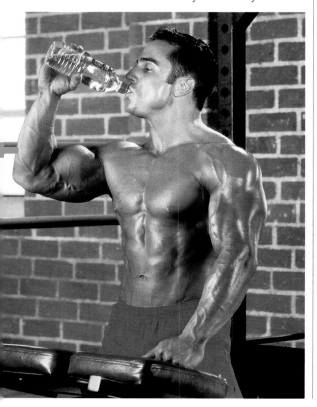

68. ALLOW YOURSELF A CHEAT DAY.

Bodybuilders often feel that cheating on their diets sabotages their goals. The solution? Schedule a little cheating, such as allowing yourself a hamburger on the weekend. Likewise, a small piece of cheesecake after dinner won't destroy your physique. In fact, it may help it in the long run: By cheating in moderation, you maintain your sanity and give yourself a much-deserved reward.

69. DON'T OBSESS ABOUT CALORIES.

Some trainees weigh every mouthful of food, calculating every fraction of a gram and every calorie. The problem with that strategy is that it's still only an approximation. A better way is to learn to use internal and external cues such as hunger, your appearance in the mirror, bodyfat tests and scales. These will give you more valuable information than merely weighing your food.

70. KEEP TRACK OF CALORIES.

On the other hand, calories *always* count, and you can't add bodyweight (good or bad) unless you take in more calories than you burn. You should get in about 18–22 calories per pound of bodyweight per day to put on quality mass, but don't let it consume your life. Learn to estimate instead of obsess.

71. CASEIN BETWEEN MEALS.

For hardgainers, it's often difficult to consume enough calories every day to promote adequate gains. What you eat can have a major impact on your hunger levels and ability to eat big. Consuming 20–40 grams of casein protein in shake form between meals can help you get in adequate protein and calories without filling you up and limiting what you eat at your next meal. Research shows that casein doesn't boost levels of hunger-blunting hormones the way whey protein does.

72. **PLAN AND PREPARE MEALS AHEAD OF TIME.** Time can be the great enemy of bodybuilding nutrition. Eating six meals a day is time-consuming, and preparing that many meals is even more so. Learn to prepare several meals at once. Find foods that are palatable and take prepared meals along with you. That way you aren't at the mercy of fast food or a schedule that doesn't allow for a break.

73. **EAT LIKE A BODYBUILDER IN RESTAURANTS.** When you eat out, you don't have to automatically go off your bodybuilding diet. Order simple meals to your specifications. Focus on meat dishes such as chicken breast or lean red meats without sauces. Order vegetables and salads as sides instead of fatty or starchy alternatives.

74. **LEARN TO READ LABELS.** Just because a particular food is bodybuilding-friendly doesn't mean it measures up once it has been packaged. Take peanut butter, for example. Low-fat varieties often contain the same number of calories as regular versions. For every fat calorie that's removed, a sugar calorie is added — and that is a bad tradeoff for bodybuilders. Learn to read labels so you know exactly what you're getting.

75. **LEARN TO SUBSTITUTE.** Ideal bodybuilding foods won't always be available, and some lifters get stressed when they're forced to eat foods off their diets or nothing at all. Interestingly, the stress itself is probably more harmful to your physique than the food. Make the best of the situation and eat to satisfy your hunger. You can always be more rigorous with your diet later on.

76. **SLOW DOWN AT NIGHT.** Before bed, you need to protect your muscles from the attack that occurs during the night. Since your body turns to your muscles for fuel while you sleep, you need to give it an alternate protein source. Taking 20–40 grams of casein protein or eating some cottage cheese will provide the long-lasting protein your body needs to protect your muscle overnight.

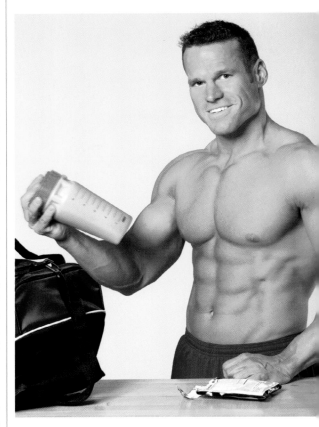

SUPPLEMENTATION

77. **TAKE GLUTAMINE FOUR TIMES A DAY.** Many bodybuilders take glutamine, but not all of them take it as often as they should. M&F considers glutamine to be a very effective supplement. Its effects are subtle at first, aiding in digestion and strengthening your immune system, then leading to quicker recovery from the stress of training. Take 5–10 grams of this amino acid with breakfast, before and after workouts, and before bed.

78. **TAKE CREATINE PRE- AND POSTWORKOUT.** Creatine can be taken any time of day, but the most effective times are before and after you train, along with protein and carbs. Research confirms that those who take creatine at these times experience gains in muscle and strength significantly higher than those who take creatine at other times of day.

79. **TAKE A MULTIVITAMIN EVERY DAY.** The limitations of a bodybuilding diet often don't provide athletes with all the vitamins, minerals and nutrients they need, especially if they give short shrift to vegetables and fruits. Since bodybuilders have greater nutrient needs than the average person, taking a multivitamin every day can ensure that you get all the nutrients you need for optimal gains.

80. **SUPPLEMENT VITAMINS C AND E.** Of all vitamins, C and E are the two most important to supplement. Both are antioxidants that fight free radicals and assist in your recovery from training. Take 1–2 grams of vitamin C and 400–800 IU of vitamin E every day.

81. **USE ZMA.** ZMA is a combination of zinc and magnesium aspartate plus vitamin B_6 that has been shown to increase testosterone and insulinlike growth factor-1, as well as boost strength and power. Take ZMA shortly before bedtime, preferably on an empty stomach for best results.

82. **SOMETHING'S FISHY.** Taking 1–3 grams of fish oil twice a day with meals is one of the smartest things a bodybuilder can do. Fish oil not only is beneficial to your heart health but it enhances joint recovery, boosts fat loss and aids muscle growth as well.

83. **BRANCH OUT.** Branched-chain amino acids (BCAAs) are comprised of three aminos — leucine, isoleucine and valine — that are most critical for muscle recovery and growth. That's because they boost muscle protein synthesis and even blunt levels of the catabolic hormone cortisol. Go with 5–10 grams of BCAAs in the morning, and before and after workouts.

84. **BOOST IT.** Using a nitric oxide (NO) booster containing arginine will help increase muscle mass and strength because NO helps regulate muscle growth and dilates blood vessels. Greater blood-vessel dilation promotes blood flow, which allows more blood — along with more oxygen, nutrients and anabolic hormones — to be delivered to the muscles. This gives you more energy and bigger pumps to carry you through your intense workouts as well as better recovery and growth afterward. Choose an NO booster that provides at least 3–5 grams of arginine, and take it as soon as you wake up in the morning and then again 30–45 minutes before workouts on an empty stomach.

85. **GET CAFFEINATED.** Before workouts, a 200–400-mg dose of caffeine will boost your training intensity as well as your muscle strength. Caffeine has been shown in numerous studies to increase endurance and strength during workouts and to blunt muscle pain, which can help you train with more intensity.

SPECIFIC TRAINING TIPS

86. **INCLINE TO BUILD YOUR CHEST.** Performing bench presses at a 30-degree incline is the No. 1 pec-builder. Bench to build your chest, not to press more weight. Often, the bench press turns into an ego exercise because lifters care more about how much weight they can lift. Instead, concentrate on the feeling in your chest. Feel the stretch in your pecs as you lower the weight, and press it up using your chest strength, not your shoulders.

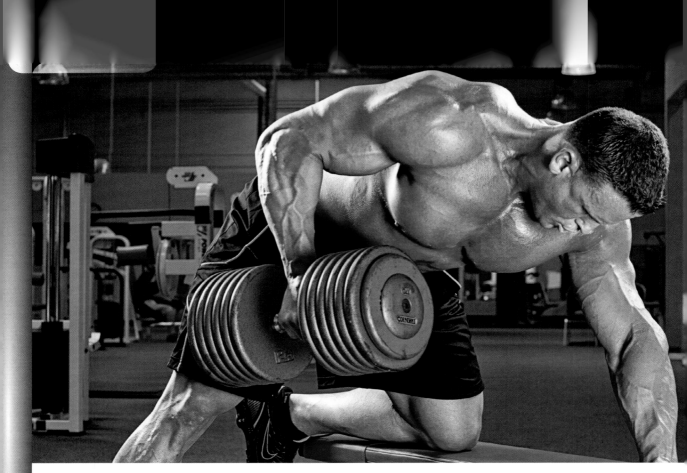

87. PERFORM FLYE MOVEMENTS WITH MODERATE WEIGHTS.

As with other chest exercises, lifters tend to use the heaviest weight possible on flyes. Yet this often recruits your shoulders into the movement. Choose a weight that allows you to feel a deep stretch across your pecs. Try dropping 10 pounds and slowing each rep, but don't increase the quantity.

88. SQUAT WITH PROPER FORM.

Too many bodybuilders think the purpose of squatting is to put as much weight as possible across their backs. Instead, try to stimulate as much muscle growth as possible in your quads, hamstrings and glutes by using a weight that allows you to squat with proper form. Keep your back tight, holding its natural curvature throughout the movement. Descend, stretching your glutes and hamstrings, and press back up through your heels. Now that's a squat.

89. HAVE A SPOTTER WHEN SQUATTING.

Due to the heavy load and the mechanics of the exercise, you should always have a spotter — preferably two — when performing to-the-max squats. This can help you power through an extra rep and ensure your personal safety.

90. INCORPORATE BOTH SEATED AND STANDING CALF RAISES.

Many bodybuilders bomb their calves with five or more sets of either standing or seated calf raises, but a better strategy is to include 2–3 sets of each. Seated calf raises target the soleus while standing calf raises target the gastrocnemius. For complete calf development, you need to target both of these muscles.

91. MAKE DEADLIFTS A PART OF YOUR TRAINING.

Too often deadlifts are considered just a powerlifter's exercise. This myth needs to be put to rest. When performed correctly, deadlifts are an excellent bodybuilding exercise. This compound move builds the entire body better than any other single exercise (even squats!). If you use strict form, deadlifts can help build your upper and lower back, abs, glutes and legs. They also increase your overall strength, making you stronger for other movements.

92. GO HEAVY ON BARBELL ROWS.
This is an out-and-out mass-builder for the back, but you must be able to handle as much weight as possible while still maintaining strict form. Rely on the overload principle with 8–12 reps to shock the muscles into growth and add density to your entire back.

93. ADD A SUPINATING MOVEMENT FOR BICEPS.
When you supinate (turn your wrist out) at the top of the movement in a dumbbell curl, you take your biceps through its full range of motion, helping to develop the muscle more fully. Supinate, then squeeze, at the top of each rep.

94. WARM UP THOROUGHLY FOR DELT TRAINING.
A proper warm-up routine is necessary for all bodyparts, but this is especially true for the injury-prone shoulder joints. Always warm up with a light series of lateral, front and bent-over raises. One set of each with 20 reps increases blood flow to and flexibility in the target zone, decreasing your risk of injury.

95. USE PROPER FORM WITH LATERAL RAISES.
For many, the goal with lateral raises seems to be to swing the weights up. Instead, your objective should be to feel a contraction in your middle delts at the top of the movement. The weight should be moderate enough that you can also control the rep cadence as you lower the weights.

96. USE DUMBBELL SHRUGS TO BUILD YOUR TRAPS.
Dumbbells offer several distinct advantages over barbells to bring up the traps. The principal benefits are a fuller range of motion and a "squeeze" that will help improve all aspects of the trapezius musculature.

FINALLY...

97. KEEP LEARNING.
This is no sales hype: Continue to read M&F. Every month, it's packed full of practical and cutting-edge training and dietary strategies you can use immediately to build muscle.

98. TRI HARDER.
Incorporate both pressing and strict extension exercises to hit all of the fibers in your triceps muscles. For example, combining the close-grip bench press with the cable pushdown makes for a great triceps-shredding workout that will produce results.

99. ABSOLUTE CONTRACTION.
Abs are a surprisingly long muscle group and need to be worked from both the top (with crunches) and bottom (reverse crunches) for maximum development. As an added kick, be sure to rotate your pelvis and round your back during each crunch.

100. FEED NOCTURNALLY.
For extra calories and a growth boost at night, down a protein shake any time you wake up to use the bathroom. This will help pulse your amino-acid levels and ensure optimal anabolism.

101. SEEK PUSHBACK.
To fully activate your lats, don't think about pulling with your hands, a situation in which the arms end up doing much of the work. Instead, think about pushing with your elbows — driving them like pistons back behind you — and you'll feel the benefits immediately. Over time, this will help you build more back mass.

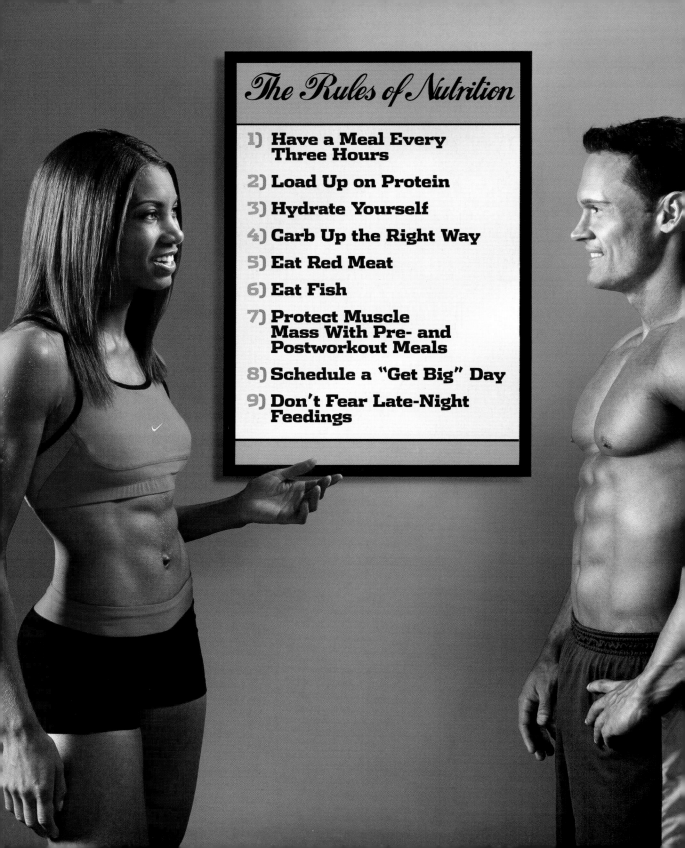

The Rules of Nutrition

1) **Have a Meal Every Three Hours**

2) **Load Up on Protein**

3) **Hydrate Yourself**

4) **Carb Up the Right Way**

5) **Eat Red Meat**

6) **Eat Fish**

7) **Protect Muscle Mass With Pre- and Postworkout Meals**

8) **Schedule a "Get Big" Day**

9) **Don't Fear Late-Night Feedings**

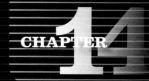

CHAPTER 14

NINE RULES OF NUTRITION

NEVER IGNORE THE IMPORTANCE DIET PLAYS IN ACHIEVING A GREAT PHYSIQUE. THESE NINE NUTRITIONAL GUIDELINES WILL LAY YOUR FOUNDATION FOR MUSCLE GROWTH

Bodybuilding is all about simplifying things. With the dedication and effort required to stay muscular and lean, the last thing you need is for the details to be overly confusing. Take your diet, for example. We could go on and on about fat-soluble vs. water-soluble vitamins, the different types of saccharides and all the intricacies of gluconeogenesis, but what would be the point? It would just complicate the matter and get you no closer to the body you want. So let's break it down to the nuts and bolts, to just the vital information you really need to build more muscle and become leaner than ever before.

The key is a series of rules, a list we call the 9 Rules of Nutrition. Follow all nine and not only will you not be bogged down with scientific jargon but you'll also be well on your way to a bigger upper body, better abs and a massive set of wheels. How's that for simple?

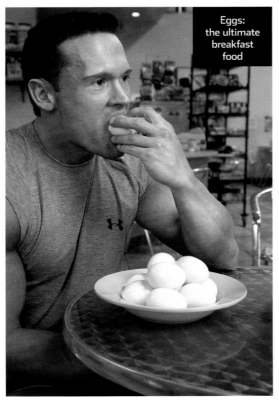

Eggs: the ultimate breakfast food

1 HAVE A MEAL EVERY THREE HOURS

Mass-building boils down to nutrient delivery, and nothing beats eating every 2–3 hours, which works out to 6–8 meals a day. Frequent feedings ensure a constant influx of protein, carbohydrates and essential fatty acids required to maintain an anabolic state. Following the three-hour rule, you should **eat at least the same amount and up to twice as many carbohydrates as protein at most meals,** along with a smaller amount of healthy fats at most meals (more on specific macronutrient intake in later rules). Because you're eating every three hours, don't overstuff yourself; keeping each meal relatively small enhances nutrient absorption while simultaneously allowing you to sidestep gains in bodyfat.

"Eating smaller, more frequent meals creates an environment inside the body in which blood sugar levels don't elevate and drop as drastically as when you eat fewer larger meals," says Justin Harris, NPC amateur bodybuilder and nutrition consultant. "Elevated blood sugar levels cause the body to increase insulin production in an attempt to store that sugar for later. When insulin is present, fat-burning is blunted. Lowered insulin levels and steady blood amino acid levels (a product of eating relatively small, frequent meals throughout the day) help fight against this situation."

2 LOAD UP ON PROTEIN

A meal should never go by without a sufficient amount of protein being consumed. To maximize muscle-building, you'll need to **consume at least 1 gram of protein per pound of bodyweight per day.** (This means 200 grams of protein daily for a 200-pound person.) In order to provide your muscles with a continuous influx of amino acids — the building blocks of protein — throughout the day, you'll divide your daily protein by the number of meals you consume. For example, if you eat six meals per day, 200 grams of protein

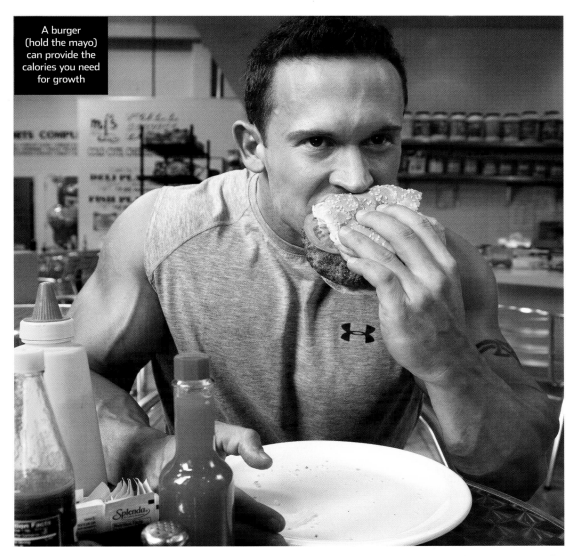

A burger (hold the mayo) can provide the calories you need for growth

divided by six meals would mean at least 30–40 grams of protein per meal.

Your main protein sources should be lean animal sources, such as chicken, beef, turkey, fish, eggs and dairy (more on red meat and fish in later rules), and, as with your training regimen, variety is crucial. Sticking to the same one or two protein sources each day may not be as effective as mixing it up and including the widest array of protein sources available. "There's a phenomenon in the body called the *all or nothing principle*, in which all amino acids must be available for proper utilization of digested protein," Harris says. "Many proteins can be made by the body; those that cannot are called essential amino acids and must be derived from nutritional sources. You'll need to mix various sources of protein to ensure that all essential amino acids are consumed."

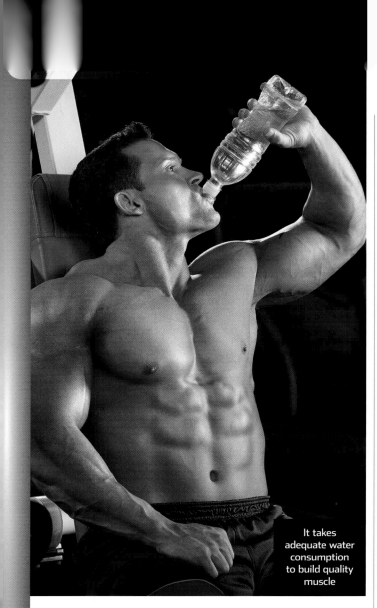

It takes adequate water consumption to build quality muscle

consultant to three-time Mr. Olympia Jay Cutler and author of *Championship Bodybuilding and Everything You Need to Know About Fat Loss* (available at nutramedia.com). "This allows the muscles to maintain a positive nitrogen balance, which directly impacts muscle growth."

And if you're supplementing with creatine, glutamine and BCAAs (more on that in Chapter 15), your muscles will have a greater capacity to store water, because when muscle cells are stocked with these nutrients, more water is actually drawn into the muscles. **Consume at least 1 gallon of water every day, and drink around 8 ounces of water every 15–20 minutes during training.**

4 CARB UP THE RIGHT WAY

When it comes to carbs, too few can shortchange your gains in mass and too many can transform you into a bulked-up softie. A good rule of thumb is to **consume 2–3 grams of carbohydrates per pound of bodyweight per day when trying to add mass.** And as with protein, you'll want to divide this between however many meals you eat daily, with the exception of two times during the day: breakfast and your postworkout meal.

"These are two times when the body is somewhat inefficient at manufacturing bodyfat from carbohydrates, so feel free to bump up your carb intake at these times of day," Aceto says. "Breakfast and the postworkout meal are also vital in aiding muscle growth because the higher carb content boosts one of the anabolic hormones responsible for driving nutrients into muscles, thereby producing a favorable hormonal environment that kick-starts recovery."

At most meals (pre- and postworkout notwithstanding, as you'll learn in rule No. 7), you should consume slow-digesting carbs such as whole-grain breads and pastas, oatmeal, sweet potatoes, fruits and vegetables, rather than fast-digesting sources such as white breads and sweets. The former help build muscle and provide sustained energy.

3 HYDRATE YOURSELF

The importance of drinking plenty of liquids goes beyond the obvious benefits of staying hydrated; at a much deeper level, it's all about pushing more water into muscle cells. The more water that's inside muscles, the better they'll function and the greater their strength and size capacity. "The consensus in the bodybuilding community is that high water storage within muscles helps act as an anabolic factor," says Chris Aceto, nutrition

5 EAT RED MEAT

Steaks and beef patties often scare people off because of the high fat content found in many cuts. But when you're looking to build muscle, shunning red meat is the last thing you want to do: It's high in B vitamins, including B_{12}, which supports muscular endurance and growth, and yields, gram for gram, more iron, creatine and zinc than any other source of protein. These nutrients play important roles in muscle recovery and growth, so if you're sticking with chicken, turkey and protein powder, you'll likely fall short of your hypertrophy goals. "Red meat is a great slow-digesting source of protein that can aid in nitrogen retention and sustained elevation of amino acids in the blood," says Alan Aragon, MS, CSCS, a private-practice nutrition counselor in Thousand Oaks, California. "Red meat can be used for all seasons, not just mass phases." When choosing an appropriate type of red meat, **select primarily leaner cuts such as ground round and sirloin, looking for meat that's at least 93% lean.**

6 EAT FISH

A lot of bodybuilders seem to live on fowl and low-fat beef, but salmon, trout, bluefish and tuna offer advantages other sources of protein can't — namely, they're sources of omega-3 fatty acids, which can indirectly make you leaner and bigger. Omega-3s help the body make glycogen, the storage form of carbohydrates that gets socked away in muscle tissue. Glycogen is the main source of energy for training and, generally speaking, adequate levels are a marker for muscle growth and repair. Omega-3s also fight muscle inflammation in the body and spare the loss of glutamine, a vital amino acid that plays a backup role in the muscle recovery process by boosting the immune system. You don't have to go overboard, but including fish in your diet a few days a week will go a long way toward promoting lean muscle gains. All in all, don't be afraid of fat — **20%–30% of your daily calories should consist of healthy dietary fat.**

"Fish is an excellent source of protein, with an amino acid profile very beneficial to enhancing muscle growth," Harris says. "Omega-3s can increase the insulin sensitivity of the tissues, creating an environment in which less insulin is necessary to shuttle nutrients around the body, which benefits you getting leaner."

> # When you're looking to build some serious muscle, avoiding vitamin B–rich red meat is the last dietary thing you want to do

7 PROTECT MUSCLE MASS WITH PRE- AND POSTWORKOUT MEALS

The catch-22 with training is that stress hormones, namely cortisol, can run amok and blunt muscle-building to the point that getting back on track is not as simple as following the basic rules. The solution? Eating and supplementing with the right foods in the pre- and post-training meals. This is where whey protein is essential — it gets into the blood faster than any other source of protein, providing amino acids that muscles harness for growth and interfere with cortisol uptake. A slower-absorbing protein such as casein takes longer to combat cortisol levels.

Throw in some fast-acting carbs — those that digest quickly such as Gatorade, fat-free Pop-Tarts, cream of rice cereal mixed with jam or a toasted bagel — and you benefit further. These carbs, when combined with whey protein, are extremely effective at almost immediately halting muscle breakdown. According to Aragon, "sandwiching" your workout with protein and carbs causes greater protein synthesis and inhibits muscle protein breakdown. **Consume at least 20 grams of whey protein before and 40 grams after training, a slow-digesting carbohydrate (refer to rule No. 4 for the best sources) 30 minutes before training and a fast-digesting carb immediately afterward, along with your whey.** As for dietary fat, pre- and postworkout are the two times of day when you want to forgo eating foods high in fat. They'll slow the absorption of protein and carbs, which will delay the muscle recovery process.

8 SCHEDULE A "GET BIG" DAY

While eating a sound diet by implementing the steps above is the foundation for growth, **taking one out of every 7–10 days and eating far above and beyond your typical daily food intake — increasing protein, carbohydrate and overall calorie intake — can trigger new muscle growth** by driving up your body's levels of growth hormones. Some people call this a "cheat day." When you occasionally overeat, the body responds by increasing the release of naturally occurring growth agents, such as growth hormone, insulinlike growth factor-1, thyroid hormone and possibly testosterone. Since even a small boost in one or all of these can impact recovery and muscle growth, it makes sense to harness them, and temporarily eating "really big" can do just that.

"Eating relatively clean all the time can lead to boredom and compromised adherence to a bodybuilding diet," Aragon says. "Periodic spikes in calorie consumption are a great way to achieve

FEED THE MACHINE

Combine all nine rules and you get a meal plan that looks something like this. As it's merely an example of what your diet could be like for one day, feel free to substitute in different foods based on your personal preferences. Also, your daily schedule may differ from this one (which is based on a standard 9-to-5 workday), so alter accordingly.

MEAL 1: 7:30 A.M.
›› 8–10 egg whites
›› 1 whole egg
›› 1 large bowl cream of rice cereal
›› 1 small banana

MEAL 2: 10 A.M.
›› 1 1/3 cup fat-free cottage cheese
›› 1 small whole-grain bagel

MEAL 3: 1 P.M.
›› 8 oz. turkey breast
›› 1 large sweet potato

MEAL 4: 3 P.M.
›› 8 oz. chicken breast
›› 2 cups whole-wheat pasta
›› 1 cup vegetables

MEAL 5: 5 P.M. PREWORKOUT
(30–60 minutes before training)
›› 20 g whey protein mixed in water
›› 2 slices whole-grain bread

MEAL 6: POSTWORKOUT
(immediately following workout)
›› 40 g whey protein mixed in water
›› 1–2 fat-free Pop-Tarts or 16 oz. Gatorade

MEAL 7: 7:30 P.M.
›› 8 oz. salmon or 8 oz. steak
›› 1 large sweet potato

BEDTIME: 10:30 P.M.
›› 30 g casein protein mixed in water or 1 cup fat-free cottage cheese
›› 2 Tbsp. peanut butter

Consuming slow-absorbing protein and healthy fats before bedtime can help hard gainers pack on muscle

a net caloric surplus that can speed muscular growth and strength. To avoid large gains in bodyfat, make sure 'once every 7–10 days' doesn't turn into cheating on most days."

9 DON'T FEAR LATE-NIGHT FEEDINGS

In the 7–9 hours you sleep every night, your body is more or less in a fasting state, taking aminos from your muscles to fuel your brain in the absence of food — not an ideal situation if your goal is to pack on muscle. However, you can offset this by eating right before you turn in for the night. The key is eating a slow-digesting protein source along with a moderate amount of fat so amino acids feed your muscles gradually throughout the night. **At bedtime, consume approximately 30 grams of casein protein or 1 cup of low-fat cottage cheese along with 1–2 tablespoons of peanut butter, an ounce of walnuts or mixed nuts, or 2–3 tablespoons of flaxseed oil.** Casein is a slow-digesting protein (as is cottage cheese) that comes in powder form, and the healthy fats found in peanut butter, nuts and flaxseed (almost exclusively unsaturated, by the way) will help slow the absorption of protein even further.

Aceto also recommends consuming protein, and even carbs, in the middle of the night if you happen to get up to use the bathroom. "That's the perfect time to have a shake," he says. "If gaining bodyfat is no issue, have 50 grams of protein mixed with 50 grams of liquid carbs such as a meal replacement shake that contains both protein and carbs, or mix the protein in fruit juice. If you're struggling to control bodyfat, though, skip the carbs. This round-the-clock nutrient delivery will keep the body in an anabolic state."

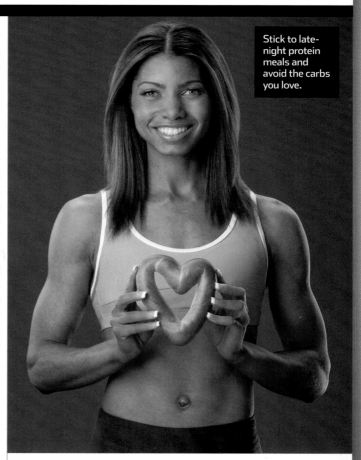

Stick to late-night protein meals and avoid the carbs you love.

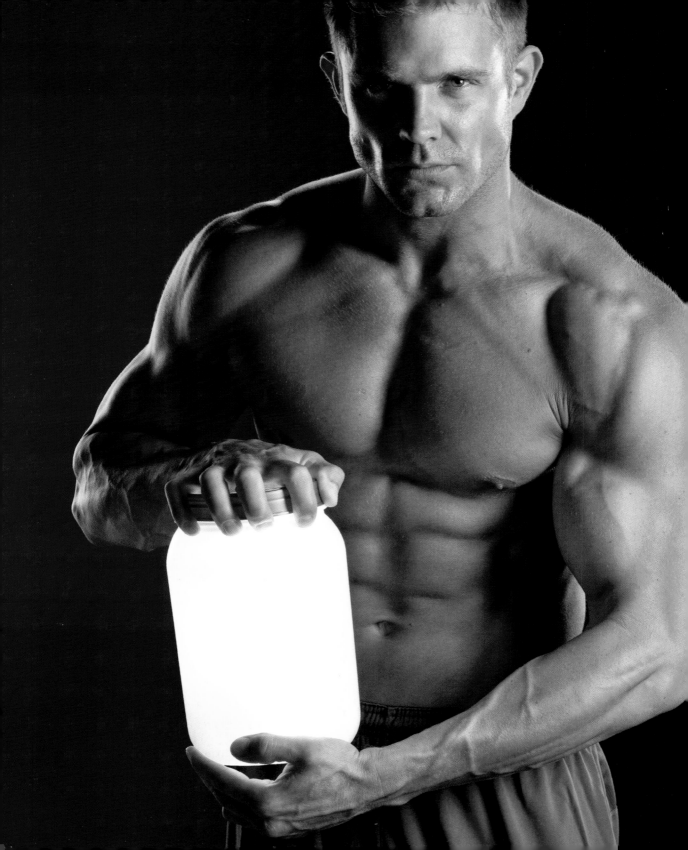

SUPPLEMENT YOUR MASS

ADD SERIOUS MUSCLE TO YOUR PHYSIQUE (UP TO 15–20 POUNDS WORTH) IN THE NEXT 12 MONTHS — ONE MAJOR MASS-BUILDING SUPPLEMENT AT A TIME

You've got a little problem (emphasis on little): You're looking to build muscle — lots of muscle. You're training like a beast and eating like one, yet you're finding that the protein shakes, creatine and nitric oxide boosters you're taking around workouts, while helpful, aren't quite delivering the mass you were hoping for. What you need to do, then, is step up your supplement plan.

We know why you've neglected to step it up — with so many different supplements on the market today, you don't know what to take, when to take it or how much of it to take. Well, leave the planning to us. Here, we give you a 12-month supplement "step-up" plan for gaining mass that starts simple and progresses steadily, bringing you to a hardcore mass supplement program one month at a time while building big time muscle along the way.

The plan starts out with the basics, then each month progresses to a new level with the addition of one or two supplements. The order the supplements are added is designed to enhance the supplements you're already taking. If you're tempted to jump right in at month 12 (to start with all 12 supplements), think again. By doing this, you won't get as much out of each supplement as you would by taking one for a while, then slowly adding the others. Our method will enhance the long-term effectiveness of the supplement stack. In fact, if

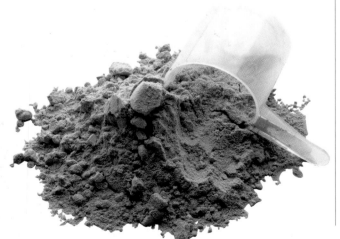

you follow the plan as outlined and adhere to a rigorous workout regimen, you can expect to add a solid 15–20 pounds of quality muscle over the course of the next year. If that's not a solution to your little problem, we don't know what is.

BASIC FOUNDATION

Cover your bases from the beginning by taking the elemental mass-gaining supplements that have proved effective by both researchers and top-level bodybuilders alike.

MONTH 1

Whey protein It gets no simpler than starting out your supplement plan with whey protein, the golden boy of protein powders. Research shows that this fast-digesting protein rich in branched-chain amino acids boosts muscle growth, especially when used around workouts. It also contains peptides that increase blood flow to the muscles. When you take whey before workouts, it helps deliver more oxygen, more nutrients and more anabolic hormones to your muscles, which provides you with more energy during workouts, an enhanced muscle pump and better muscle recovery and growth after training.

Mass Prescription: Take 20 grams of whey protein (mixed in water) within 30 minutes before each workout and another 40 grams within 30 minutes after working out.

MONTH 2

ZMA This combination of zinc and magnesium aspartate plus vitamin B_6 can help boost testosterone and insulinlike growth factor-1 levels, while blunting levels of the catabolic hormone cortisol, all of which support muscle growth and strength gains. Numerous studies have shown that both zinc and magnesium achieve those goals for athletes. And how can simple minerals work in this manner? Because hard training depletes zinc and magnesium, so supplementing with this precise combination will bring levels back up for optimal gains.

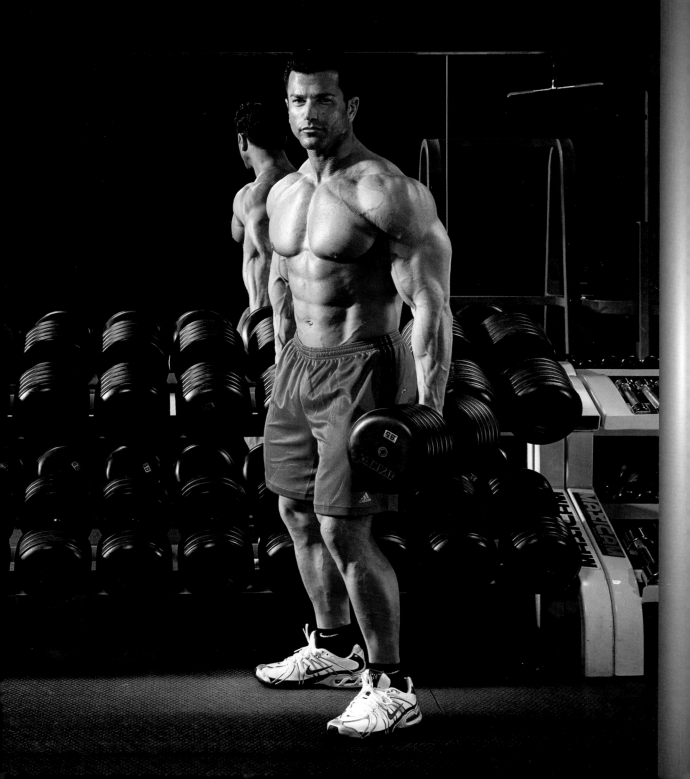

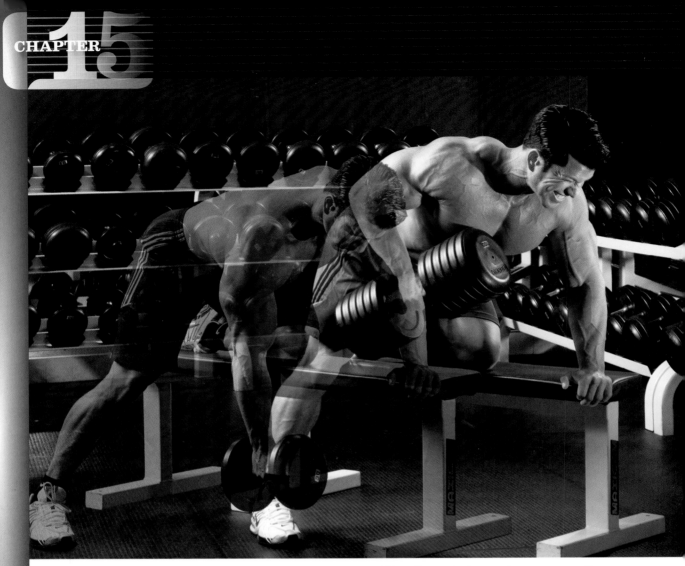

Mass Prescription: Choose a ZMA product that provides about 30 mg of zinc, 450 mg of magnesium and about 10.5 mg of vitamin B$_6$, and take it 30–60 minutes before bedtime without any food or calcium (dairy) — this will enhance its uptake and utilization and give you better quality sleep for optimal recovery.

MONTH 3
Creatine Made from the amino acids arginine, glycine and methionine, creatine is the proven thoroughbred of bodybuilding supplements. Hundreds of studies support its effectiveness, with reports of gains in strength of over 10% and gains in muscle over 10 pounds.

Mass Prescription: Take 2–5 grams of creatine in the form of creatine monohydrate, creatine malate, creatine ethyl ester or creatine alpha-ketoglutarate within 30 minutes before workouts, and take another 2–5 grams within 30 minutes after training.

UPPING THE ANTE
Once you've created a solid supplement foundation with whey, ZMA and creatine, it's time to step up your supplement plan by progressively adding the following three supplements to supercharge the benefits of the first three.

MONTH 4

Casein Whey makes up just 20% of the protein in milk, while casein makes up the remaining 80%. The latter, however, has always been considered inferior to whey, which is mostly due to its slow rate of digestion. This factor makes it valuable as a pre-bedtime snack to prevent muscle breakdown during sleep, but casein has long been avoided by bodybuilders around workout time. However, that's all changed, thanks to new research. Now we know that when it's taken after workouts, casein boosts muscle protein synthesis similar to whey. Research even shows that when trained lifters replace some of the whey in their postworkout shake with casein, they gain significantly more muscle mass than those not adding casein to whey.

Mass Prescription: After workouts, supercharge your postworkout whey shake by replacing 10–20 grams of whey with casein in the form of micellar casein, calcium caseinate, sodium caseinate or potassium caseinate.

*Strong Suit: During this month, add another 20- to 40-gram dose of whey as soon as you wake in the morning.

MONTH 5

BCAAs Branched-chain amino acids — leucine, isoleucine and valine — are hands down the most critical amino acids for repairing and building muscle. They stimulate muscle protein synthesis, which leads to muscle growth, and they also blunt the catabolic hormone cortisol. Taking BCAAs before workouts is important because muscles use these aminos for fuel, helping to prevent fatigue during workouts. And although whey is rich in BCAAs, boosting your postworkout whey shake with extra BCAAs will give you additional gains in both strength and muscle mass. In fact, preliminary research from our own Weider Research Group shows that trained lifters taking BCAAs around workout time experienced significantly greater gains in muscle mass and strength as compared to those taking a placebo.

Mass Prescription: Take 5 gram of BCAAs with your breakfast, preworkout and postworkout shakes. Look for BCAA products that provide leucine at a ratio of 2:1 per dose of isoleucine and valine. For example, a 5-gram dose of BCAAs should provide 2.5 grams of leucine, 1.25 grams of isoleucine and 1.25 grams of valine.

MONTH 6

NO Booster Nitric oxide is a ubiquitous molecule, meaning it's found throughout the body and is involved in multiple processes — namely the dilation of blood vessels, wherein they become wider in diameter, allowing more blood flow to your muscles to deliver more oxygen, nutrients and anabolic hormones. Because NO works through a different mechanism than whey peptides to increase blood flow, taking NO boosters has an additive effect that leads to even greater energy during workouts, a bigger muscle pump and even better muscle recovery and growth after training. NO will also boost the benefits of a ZMA supplement, as NO works to free up zinc in the body so that it can perform its work. Although some bodybuilders think NO boosters actually provide NO, they in fact supply NO precursors, such as the amino acids arginine and citrulline, as well as ingredients that help convert these aminos into NO, such as Pycnogenol.

Mass Prescription: Take an NO booster that provides 3–5 grams of arginine in the form of L-arginine, arginine alpha-ketoglutarate, arginine ethyl ester or arginine malate in the morning before breakfast, about 30–60 minutes before workouts and 30–60 minutes before bedtime.

THE NEXT LEVEL

Once you've stepped up your supplement regimen, it's time to take it to the next level with these three hardcore mass and strength supplements that will keep your gains coming by not only providing their own unique benefits, but by enhancing the benefits of the six supplements you're already taking.

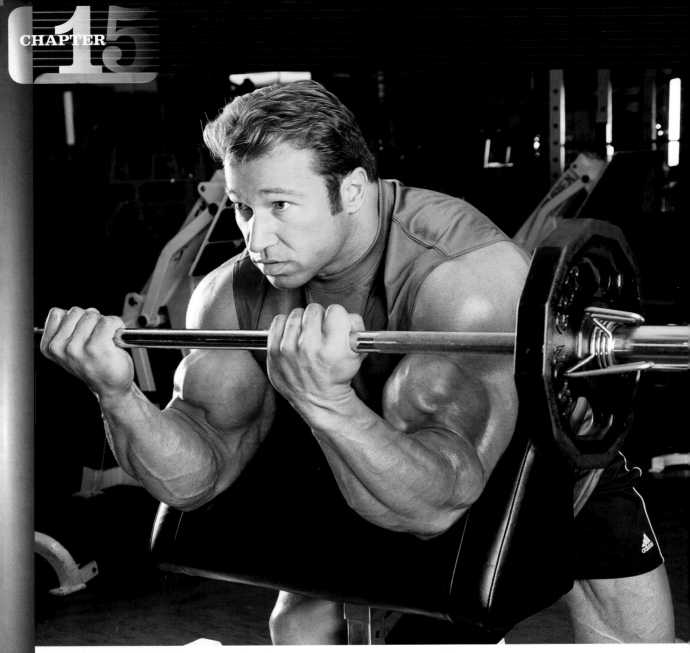

MONTH 7

Caffeine This is one of our favorite preworkout supplements, and not just because of the quick pick-me-up caffeine supplies, but because numerous research studies show that it enhances workouts. Caffeine provides the needed drive and energy for high-intensity training, which will further boost the energy aid you're getting from whey, BCAAs and NO boosters. Caffeine has also been shown to immediately increase muscle strength, which will further enhance the strength gains you'll experience from creatine. Moreover, caffeine blunts muscle pain during workouts so that you can take your training to failure, and beyond, for maximum gains in muscle size.

Mass Prescription: Take 200–400 mg of caffeine in the form of a supplement about an hour before workouts. M&F recommends a supplement rather

12-STEP MASS-BUILDING PROGRAM

Follow this month-to-month Supplement Step-Up plan for maximal mass and strength gains.

MONTH	SUPPLEMENT	MONTH	SUPPLEMENT
1	Whey protein (20 g within 30 minutes before workouts and another 40 g within 30 minutes after workouts)	7	Whey protein, ZMA, creatine, BCAAs and NO booster, as in month 6, plus . . . Casein (10–20 g added to your postworkout whey shake and 20–40 g immediately before bedtime) and Caffeine (200–400 mg about an hour before workouts)
2	Whey protein, as in month 1, plus . . . ZMA (one dose of 30 mg of zinc, 450 mg of magnesium and 10.5 mg of B6 30–60 minutes before bedtime on an empty stomach)	8	Whey protein, casein, ZMA, creatine, BCAAs, NO booster and caffeine, as in month 7, plus . . . Vitargo S2 (70 g mixed into postworkout shakes)
3	Whey protein and ZMA, as in month 2, plus . . . Creatine (2–5 g within 30 minutes before and after workouts)	9	Whey protein, casein, ZMA, creatine, BCAAs, NO booster, caffeine and Vitargo S2, as in month 8, plus . . .Beta-alanine (1 g with preworkout and postworkout shakes)
4	ZMA and creatine, as in month 3, plus . . . Whey protein (20–40 g first thing in the morning; 20 g within 30 minutes before workouts; and another 40 g within 30 minutes after workouts) and Casein (10–20 g with your postworkout whey shake)	10	Whey protein, casein, ZMA, creatine, BCAAs, NO booster, caffeine and Vitargo S2, as in month 9, plus . . . Beta-alanine (2 g with preworkout and postworkout shakes) and Carnitine (1–1.5 g with breakfast, preworkout and postworkout shakes and nighttime meals)
5	Whey protein, casein, ZMA and creatine, as in month 4, plus . . . BCAAs (5 g with breakfast, preworkout and postworkout shakes)	11	Whey protein, casein, ZMA, creatine, BCAAs, NO booster, caffeine, Vitargo S2 and beta-alanine, as in month 10, plus . . . Carnitine (2–3 g with breakfast, preworkout and postworkout shakes and nighttime meals) and Betaine (1,250 mg twice a day with meals)
6	Whey protein, casein, ZMA, creatine and BCAAs, as in month 5, plus . . . NO booster (one dose that provides 3–5 g of arginine in the morning before breakfast, 30–60 minutes before workouts and 30–60 minutes before bedtime)	12	Whey protein, casein, ZMA, creatine NO booster, caffeine, Vitargo S2, beta-alanine, carnitine and betaine, as in month 11, plus . . . BCAAs (10 g with breakfast, preworkout and postworkout shakes) and Forskolin (20–50 mg two or three times per day on an empty stomach)

CAFFEINE

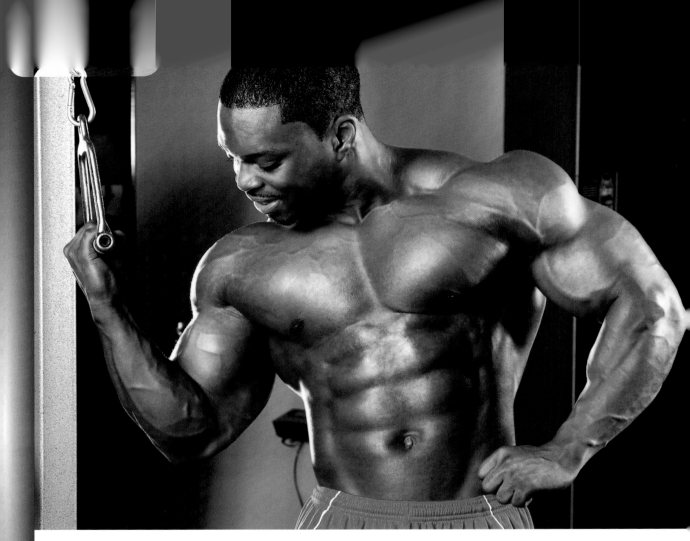

than coffee because the caffeine content of coffee can vary widely. Also, studies tend to show that coffee doesn't enhance performance as well as caffeine supplements.

*Strong Suit: This month, add a 20- to 40-gram casein shake to your diet (be sure to use a casein protein product that contains micellar casein), drinking it immediately before bedtime. Casein is a slow-burning protein that will help stave off the breakdown of muscle that occurs while you sleep.

MONTH 8

Vitargo S2 Vitargo is a patented carbohydrate supplement supported by ample clinical research showing that it moves through the stomach more than twice as fast as typical sugars, such as those found in sports drinks. This means it gets into your bloodstream much faster than any other carb, resulting in an incredible spike in the anabolic hormone insulin, which will help deliver those carbs (as well as the amino acids and creatine in your postworkout shake) into your muscle fibers. The new form of Vitargo, called Vitargo S2, mixes better into fluids than the older version of Vitargo.

Mass Prescription: Combine 70 grams of Vitargo S2 with your postworkout shake.

MONTH 9

Beta-Alanine This amino acid gets combined with the amino acid histidine in the body to form carnosine. Muscles with higher levels of carnosine have greater strength and endurance, as carnosine increases the muscle's ability to contract with more force and to do so for longer without fatiguing. Studies confirm that athletes taking beta-alanine experience increased muscle strength and endurance. Research also shows that beta-alanine enhances creatine's ability to stimulate muscle growth, as trained lifters taking beta-alanine plus creatine gained significantly more muscle mass than those taking just creatine.

Mass Prescription: Take 1 gram of beta-alanine with your preworkout and postworkout shakes.

OVER THE TOP

Once you've taken your supplement plan to the next level, it's time to take it over the top with these final three supplements that will ramp up testosterone levels and further boost your muscle mass and strength gains throughout the rest of the year.

MONTH 10

Carnitine This supplement can enhance muscle growth through a number of mechanisms, all of which are supported by clinical research. For starters, carnitine increases blood flow to muscles, which means it further boosts the effects provided by NO boosters and whey protein. In addition, carnitine increases testosterone levels after workouts and the amount of testosterone receptors inside muscle cells (known as androgen receptors), which allows more testosterone to stimulate further muscle growth.

Mass Prescription: Take 1–1.5 grams of carnitine in the form of L-carnitine, acetyl-L-carnitine, glycine propionyl-L-carnitine or L-carnitine-L-tartrate with breakfast, preworkout shakes, postworkout shakes and nighttime meals.

*Strong Suit: In month 10, increase your beta-alanine dose to 2 grams with your preworkout and postworkout shakes.

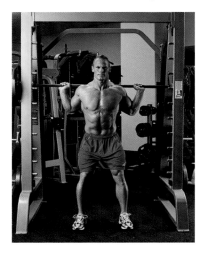

MONTH 11

Betaine Also known as trimethylglycine, this metabolite of choline can lead to even higher levels of creatine because it helps the body to produce its own creatine. Recent research showed that athletes taking betaine experienced 25% greater gains in muscle strength than those taking a placebo. This means that betaine further enhances the strength gains from creatine and beta-alanine. Betaine also enhances joint recovery, which can help you maintain training intensity and avoid injury.

Mass Prescription: Take 1,250 mg of betaine twice a day with meals.

*Strong Suit: Increase carnitine dosages this month to 2–3 grams with breakfast, preworkout shakes, postworkout shakes and nighttime meals.

MONTH 12

Forskolin This active ingredient from the herb Coleus forskohlii works to boost testosterone levels via activation of the enzyme adenylate cyclase, which ramps up testosterone production by the testes. Research shows that young males taking forskolin for 12 weeks experienced an increase in the amount of free testosterone, the active form of testosterone that provides anabolic properties upon binding to its receptor in muscle cells. Therefore, forskolin works synergistically with carnitine to kick your body into an even higher anabolic state.

Mass Prescription: Look for a Coleus forskohlii supplement that's standardized to provide 20–50 mg of forskolin and take it two or three times per day on an empty stomach.

*Strong Suit: This month, increase BCAA dosages to 10 grams — taken with breakfast, preworkout shakes and postworkout shakes.

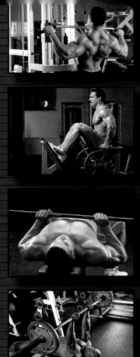

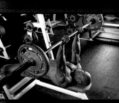

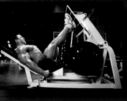

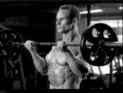

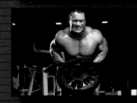

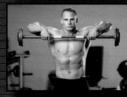

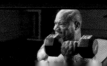

INDEX OF EXERCISES

Cable Crunch

Kneel a couple of feet in front of cable weight stack with a rope attached to a high-pulley cable. Grasp the ends of the rope and hold it at the sides of your head. Begin slightly bent over, then contract your abs to lower your torso toward the floor. As with the crunch, the range of motion here is slight; your head shouldn't reach the floor. The key is a full contraction of the abs.

Crunch

Lie faceup on the floor with your knees and hips bent about 90 degrees, feet in the air, and either cross your arms over your chest or place your hands lightly behind your head. Contract your abs to lift your shoulder blades off the floor, then lower slowly. The range of motion is very short; the goal is to press your lower back into the floor to bring your sternum closer to your pelvis.

Exercise-Ball Crunch

Lie faceup on a ball and place your feet on the floor with your knees at around a 90-degree angle. Pick a point on the ceiling and focus on that to help steady your spine and neck. Contract your abs to lift your shoulder blades off the ball, then lower slowly. The closer together your feet are, the less stable your position and thus the more difficult the exercise. You can also increase difficulty by sitting farther back on the ball.

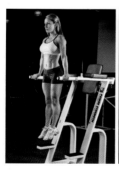 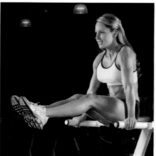

Hanging Leg Raise

Hang from a pull-up bar or vertical bench with your legs straight and perpendicular to the floor. Keeping your knees extended but not locked out, raise your legs in front of you until they're parallel to the floor. Concentrate on contracting your abs, not your hip flexors, throughout the movement. Slowly lower your legs back to the hanging position.

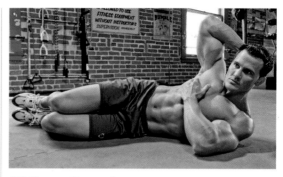

Oblique Crunch

Lie on your left side, legs on top of each other with your knees bent, using your right hand to cup your head. Crunch up as high as you can, keeping the move in the lateral plane as much as possible to emphasize the obliques, and lower under control. Repeat for reps, then switch to your right side.

Reverse Crunch

Lie faceup on the floor with your hands at your sides or under your glutes. Begin with your legs extended and your feet a few inches off the floor, suspended in the air to put tension on your abs. Contract your abs to slowly raise your legs, keeping them straight, until they're roughly perpendicular to the floor. (As with the hanging leg raise, your abs are the focus, not your hip flexors.) Slowly lower your legs back to the start position without letting your feet touch the floor.

Double Crunch

Lie on the floor with your hands cupped gently behind your head and your legs almost completely straight and raised a few inches off the floor. Simultaneously bring your knees to your torso while crunching your upper body toward your legs. Squeeze in the middle, then return to the start and repeat. Don't let your feet touch the floor between reps.

Russian Twist

Lie faceup on the floor and extend your arms overhead, grasping something secure. Keeping your shoulders on the floor but elevating your hips slightly, extend your legs above you and slowly lower them to the floor on the right side. Reverse to touch the floor on the left side. Add resistance by holding a medicine ball between your knees.

ABS

Pull-Up

Take a wide grip on a pull-up bar (hands outside shoulder width) and start in a hanging position, arms fully extended. Pull yourself up explosively by contracting your lats until your chin clears the bar. Slowly lower yourself to the start position.

Chin-Up

Assume a narrow grip, supinated grip (hands 12–18 inches apart and palms facing you) on a pull-up bar and start in a hanging position, arms fully extended. Pull yourself up explosively by contracting your lats until your chin clears the bar. Slowly lower yourself to the start position.

Lat Pulldown

Adjust the seat of the machine so your knees fit snugly under the pads. Grasp the bar outside shoulder width, arms fully extended overhead. Contract your lats to pull the bar down past your chin, squeeze your back muscles and slowly return the weight to the start position.

Barbell Bent-Over Row

Stand holding a barbell with a shoulder-width, overhand grip. Bend your knees slightly and lean forward at the waist so your torso is angled roughly 45 degrees to the floor; maintain this position throughout. Start with your arms extended, hanging straight down, and bend your elbows to pull the bar into your midsection. At the top of the move, squeeze your shoulder blades together for a count to fully contract your back muscles, then slowly return to the start position. For a reverse-grip bent-over row, the technique is the same, except that your hands will hold the bar in an underhand (supinated) grip.

Seated Cable Row

Sit on the bench of a cable-row station with your feet flat on the platform. Bend at your waist to grasp the attachment with both hands and sit upright (back flat, not bowed), arms extended in front of you. Bend your elbows to pull the handle straight toward your midsection by contracting your back muscles; de-emphasize the amount of work your biceps do to keep maximal tension on your back. When your hands reach your abs, squeeze your shoulder blades together and hold before slowly returning to the start.

T-Bar Row

With your feet flat on the platform of a T-bar row apparatus and your knees slightly bent, take a narrow grip on the bar and start with your arms fully extended toward the floor. Pull the weight toward your midsection by contracting your middle back muscles. When you've pulled the bar as far up as possible (as far as the weight plates will allow), slowly lower it back to the arms extended position.

One-Arm Dumbbell Row

Place one knee and the same-side hand on a flat bench, bent over at the waist. Keep your other foot on the floor beside the bench and hold a dumbbell in the same-side hand hanging straight down with your arm fully extended. Pull the weight up into your side, keeping your elbow in close. Pull your elbow as high as you can, squeezing your shoulder blades together for a full contraction, then lower.

Straight-Arm Pulldown

Stand facing a cable stack and attach a straight bar or rope handle to a high-pulley cable. Grasp the attachment with both hands and begin with your arms extended in front of you and your hands at roughly head height. (Make sure the weight isn't resting on the stack.) Contract your lats to pull the weight down toward your thighs, keeping your elbows extended to isolate your back muscles.

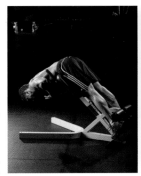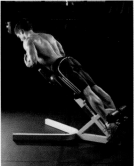

Back Extension

Secure your feet in a back-extension apparatus and allow your upper body to hang down freely, keeping your back flat. Cross your arms over your chest, squeeze your glutes and slowly raise your torso until your body forms a straight line. Slowly return the way you came.

BICEPS/FOREARMS

Barbell Curl

Stand holding a barbell in front of your thighs, arms extended and knees slightly bent to relieve pressure on your lower back. Keeping your elbows at your sides, bend them to curl the weight as high as you can. Squeeze your biceps for a count at the top, then slowly return the bar to the start position.

Dumbbell Curl

Hold a pair of dumbbells outside your thighs, palms up. Using one arm at a time, curl each dumbbell up toward your shoulder without swinging the weight or rolling your shoulder, making sure your upper arm is locked at your side. Squeeze your biceps at the top, then slowly lower to the start.

Preacher Curl

Adjust the seat of a preacher bench so the top of the pad touches your armpits. Sit down and grasp a straight bar or EZ-bar with a shoulder-width grip, arms extended but not locked out. With your upper arms flush against the pad, curl the weight as high as you can and squeeze the contraction. Lower the bar under control, again stopping just shy of locking out your elbows.

Incline Dumbbell Curl

Adjust an incline bench to 45–60 degrees and lie faceup on the bench with your feet flat on the floor. Hold a pair of dumbbells with your arms hanging straight down, palms forward. Keeping your shoulders back and upper arms fixed perpendicular to the floor, curl the dumbbells toward your shoulders. Squeeze your biceps hard at the top before slowly returning to the start position.

Machine Preacher Curl

Adjust the seat of the machine so your elbows line up with its axis of rotation. Sit down and grasp the bar with a shoulder-width grip, your arms extended but not locked out in front of you. With your upper arms flush against the pad, curl the bar as high as you can and squeeze the contraction. Lower the bar under control, stopping just shy of locking out your elbows.

Hammer Curl

Stand holding a pair of dumbbells at your sides with your wrists in a neutral position (palms facing in). Flex your elbows to curl both dumbbells up without turning your palms up — keep them in the neutral position. Squeeze your biceps and forearms at the top, then lower the weights to the start position. Hammer curls can also be performed in alternating fashion, one arm at a time.

Reverse Curl

Stand holding a straight bar or EZ-bar with a reverse grip (palms facing backward) and your arms extended straight down in front of you. Keeping your elbows in at your sides, curl the weight up, squeezing your biceps and forearms at the top, then slowly lower to the start position.

Barbell Wrist Curl

Straddle a flat bench with your feet flat on the floor. Hold a straight bar with a palms-up grip and rest the backs of your forearms on the bench with your hands past the end of it so they aren't supported. Start with your wrists extended so your knuckles point toward the floor and only your fingers hold the bar. Flex your wrists by contracting your forearm muscles to raise the bar; the range of motion is only a few inches. Squeeze your forearms for 1–2 counts at the top, then slowly return to the wrists-extended position.

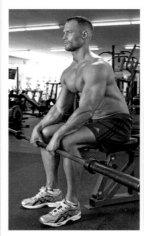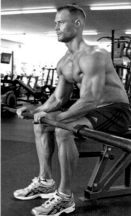

Reverse Barbell Wrist Curl

Sit at the end of a flat bench, holding a barbell with a narrow, overhand grip. Allow your forearms to rest on your quads, with only your hands extending past your knees. Curl the bar upward, squeezing your forearms, then return to the start position.

Bench Press

Lie faceup on a flat bench with a rack and grasp the barbell just outside shoulder width. Carefully lift the bar off the rack and slowly lower it toward your chest. Lightly touch the bar to your lower pecs, then forcefully press it up to an arms-extended position without locking out your elbows. The bar should be directly over your face. The path of motion here is a slight backward arc rather than a straight line up from the lower pecs.

Smith Machine Bench Press

Position a flat bench in the center of a Smith machine so that when you lower the bar, it touches your lower pecs. Lie faceup on the bench and grasp the bar outside shoulder width. Lower the bar to your chest under control, then press it back up explosively and repeat.

Flat-Bench Dumbbell Press

Lie on a flat bench and hold a set of dumbbells just above chest level with your palms facing forward and your wrists directly over your elbows. Press the dumbbells up and inward toward each other over your midchest until your elbows are almost locked out. Bring the weights back down until your elbows form 90-degree angles.

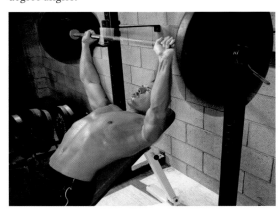

Incline Barbell Press

Lay back on a 45-degree inclined bench with a rack and grasp the bar with a slightly wider than shoulder-width grip. Start with the bar straight over your upper pecs and your arms extended but not locked out. Lower the bar to your chest, then press it up forcefully to the start position.

Incline Dumbbell Press

Lie faceup on an adjustable incline bench and start with the dumbbells just outside your shoulders. Press the weights straight above you until your elbows are extended but not locked out. Slowly return to the start position.

Decline Barbell Press

Lie faceup on a decline bench with a rack and grasp a barbell with a wider than shoulder-width grip. Unrack the weight, begin with your arms extended over you and lower the bar to your chest. After lightly touching the bar to your lower pecs, press it up to the start position without locking out your elbows.

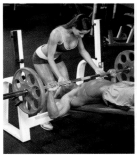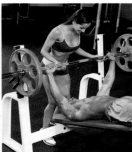

Decline Dumbbell Press

Lie faceup on a decline bench with your feet secured beneath the pads and start with the dumbbells just outside your lower pecs. Press the weights straight up until your elbows are extended but not locked out. Slowly return to the start position.

Chest Press Machine

Adjust the seat of the machine so that when placed on the handles your hands are at lower chest height. Sit with your back flat against the pad and begin with the weight off the stack to keep tension on the pecs. Press the weight away from you by contracting your chest muscles and extending your arms until your elbows are fully extended but not locked out. Keep your eyes facing forward throughout.

Flat-Bench Dumbbell Flye

Lie faceup on the bench with your feet flat on the floor. Hold a dumbbell in each hand with a neutral grip and extend your arms above your chest. Bend your elbows slightly. Slowly lower the dumbbells in

CHEST

a wide arc out to your sides. Keep your elbows locked in the slightly bent position throughout the range of motion. Stop when your elbows reach shoulder level, then contract your pecs to reverse the motion and return to the start position.

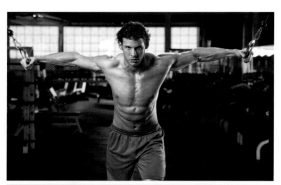

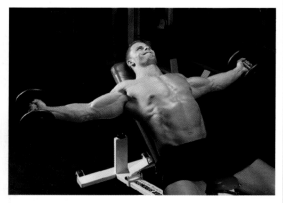

Incline Dumbbell Flye
Lie faceup on an adjustable bench set to 45 degrees, holding a pair of dumbbells over your chest with your arms extended and palms facing each other. With a slight bend in your elbows, lower the weights out in an arc to your sides until you feel a good stretch in your pecs. Contract your muscles to return the dumbbells to the start position, maintaining the slight bend in your elbows throughout.

Dip
Start by holding yourself between the bars of a dip apparatus with your arms extended. Lower yourself under control until your upper arms are parallel to the floor and you feel a good stretch in your chest, then push with your chest and triceps to lift yourself back to the start position.

Dumbbell Pullover
Place your upper back across a flat bench with your knees bent and your feet on the floor in front of you for balance. Hold one end of a dumbbell with both hands, the other end hanging down, and your arms extended with the weight over your chest. With only a slight bend in your elbows, lower the dumbbell in an arc beyond your head until you feel a stretch in your chest and lats. Pull the weight back to the start position by contracting your pecs.

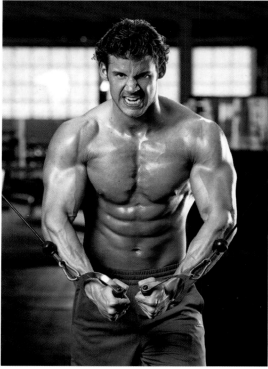

Cable Crossover
Stand in the middle of a two-sided cable station with D-handles attached to both high-pulley cables. Begin with your arms extended out to your sides and elbows slightly bent. Step forward to make sure the weights aren't resting on the stacks, then contract your pecs to pull your hands together, maintaining the slight bend in your elbows. At the end of the motion, cross your hands and squeeze your pecs for a count.

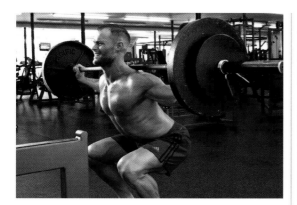

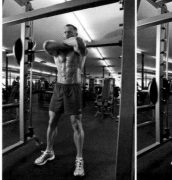
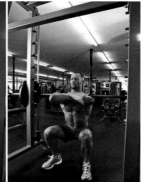

Squat (Barbell and Bodyweight)

Stand with a barbell resting across your upper traps, grasping it with your hands to keep it stable. With your feet about shoulder-width apart and head facing forward, push your chest out slightly so your back arches naturally. Squat down with the weight as if sitting in a chair, keeping your feet in full contact with the floor and maintaining the arch in your back. When your thighs reach parallel to the floor, press through your heels, extending your knees and hips to return to standing. A bodyweight squat consists of the same technique, only with no added weight via a barbell.

Barbell Front Squat

Stand inside a power rack with the barbell across your front delts and upper chest. Cross your arms over your chest to build a shelf for the bar, unrack it and step back so you clear the rack. Keep your chest up and back flat, eyes focused forward. With your abs tight, bend your knees and hips as if to sit in a chair until your thighs are well past parallel to the floor. Reverse direction by driving through your heels and pressing your hips forward.

Smith Machine Squat

Stand erect with the bar across your upper back, your feet shoulder-width apart, knees slightly bent and your toes turned out slightly. Rotate the bar to unrack it. Keeping your eyes focused forward and abs tight, bend at the knees and hips to slowly lower your body, as if sitting down in a chair. Pause when your knees reach a 90-degree angle, then forcefully drive through your heels, extending at your hips and knees until you arrive at the standing position.

Smith Machine Front Squat

Stand in a Smith machine with the bar resting across your front delts, holding it in your hands with your arms crossed over each other. Position your feet about shoulder-width apart and a foot or so in front of the bar. Face forward and push your chest out slightly so your back arches naturally. Undo the safety hooks, then squat down as if sitting in a chair, keeping your feet in full contact with the floor and maintaining the arch in your back. When your thighs reach parallel to the floor, push yourself up through your heels, extending your knees and hips, to return to the standing position.

Leg Press

Sit on a leg-press machine and place your feet hip- to shoulder-width apart on the foot platform above you. Press the weight up with your legs to a point at which your knees are extended but not locked out. Release the machine's safety catches. Lower the weight under control until your knees form 90-degree angles or slightly less. Push the weight back up explosively to the start position, again without locking out your knees at the top.

Deadlift

Stand in an open space with a loaded barbell on the floor in front of you, feet hip-width apart. Keeping your back flat and head up, bend your knees and hips to grasp the bar with a shoulder-width staggered (one palm facing forward, the other backward) grip. This is your start position. Stand up with the bar in one explosive motion by extending your knees and hips. Never round your back. Return to the start position, weight touching the floor, under control.

LEGS/HAMSTRINGS/CALVES

Dumbbell Lunge

Hold a dumbbell in each hand and stand with your feet hip-width apart and your arms down at your sides. Pull your abs in toward your spine and focus on a point on the floor a few feet in front of you. Step forward a comfortable stride length with one foot, lift the back heel, and lower your back knee straight down toward the floor. When your front thigh is parallel to the floor, press off the heel of your front foot, raising your body straight back up to the start position. Step forward and repeat with the other foot. Continue alternating legs until you've completed all the reps for one set.

Smith Machine Lunge

Stand in a Smith machine with the bar resting across your upper traps and your feet together. Unhook the latches and step a few feet forward with one foot, keeping both legs extended. Bend your front knee and drop your back knee to the floor until it's a few inches from touching. (Your front knee should not extend past your toes; if it does, step out further.) Contract the quad and glute of your front leg to press yourself back up to the standing position. Perform for desired number of reps, then switch leg positions and repeat.

Wall Squat

Place an exercise ball between your back and a wall. Begin by leaning slightly back against the ball with your legs extended and your arms at your sides. Bend your knees and lower your glutes straight down until your thighs are parallel with the floor. Extend your knees and contract your quads and glutes to return to the legs extended position without locking out your knees at the top.

Leg Extension

Adjust the seat of a leg-extension machine so that your lower back is flat against the seatback and your knees line up with the machine's axis of rotation. Begin with your legs bent 90 degrees and the weight lifted a few inches off the stack. Contract your quads to extend until your legs are completely straight. Squeeze your quads at the top, then return to the start position.

Barbell Step-Up

Select a bench or box that's 12–18 inches high. Start by standing upright with a barbell across your upper traps (as when squatting), keeping your head up and chest out for proper back alignment. Step up so that your entire foot is on the bench, then stand up, pressing into the bench and pulling your trailing leg upward. After both feet are on the bench, slowly move your trailing leg back down, emphasizing the negative motion. Maintain proper back alignment during the lift. Alternate legs every other rep, or do all your reps with one leg and then switch.

Push Press

Take a barbell from a power rack with a shoulder-width overhand grip, resting it across your upper chest, and step back. With your head up, chest out and the feet shoulder-width apart, initiate the movement by flexing your ankles, hips and knees slightly so your body descends about 4 inches. Rapidly extend your hips, knees and ankles to fully extend your body, then quickly press the bar in front of your face to elbow lockout at the top. Lower the bar back to your upper chest, bending your hips and knees slightly to cushion the weight before starting the next rep.

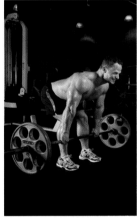 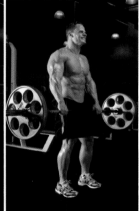

Romanian Deadlift

Stand upright, holding a barbell in front of your thighs with a shoulder-width grip. With your back flat and knees slightly bent, bend at the waist to slide the bar down your legs as you lower it straight toward the floor. Keep your knees slightly bent and your arms straight throughout the movement. When the bar reaches about mid-shin level (how far you can lower it depends on your flexibility), contract your hamstrings and glutes to pull yourself back up to the start position.

Smith Machine Romanian Deadlift

Stand upright holding the bar in front of your upper thighs with an overhand grip. Keep your feet shoulder-width apart and a slight bend in your knees. Rotate and unrack the bar. Keeping your abs pulled in tight while maintaining the natural arch in your low back, lean forward at your hips, pushing them rearward until your torso is roughly parallel to the floor. As you lean forward, keep your arms straight as the bar travels toward the bottom of the guide rods. At the bottom, keep your back flat and head neutral, then flex your hamstrings and glutes to lift your torso while pushing your hips forward until the bar reaches the start position.

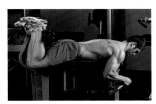

Lying Leg Curl

Adjust the machine so the roller pad fits on the backs of your ankles. Lie facedown and grasp the handles. Start with your legs straight and the weight lifted a few inches off the stack. Bend your knees to curl the roller pad toward your glutes. Squeeze your hamstrings for a count at the top and slowly lower to the start position.

Seated Leg Curl

Adjust the seat so your knees line up with the machine's axis of rotation. Sit squarely in the machine, placing the backs of your ankles on the rollers and securing the pad across your lower quads. Begin with your legs extended, then contract your hamstrings to flex your knees as far as possible. Hold for a count at the bottom, then slowly return to the start position.

Exercise Ball Leg Curl

Lie on your back on the floor with your hands next to your hips and your heels on top of an exercise ball. Pull in your abs and tighten your glutes to lift your body into a straight line from shoulders to heels. Keeping your hips off the floor, bend your knees and contract your hamstrings to pull the ball toward your glutes. Keeping your abs tight, roll the ball back out and repeat for reps.

Standing Calf Raise

Step onto the platform so only the balls of your feet and toes touch it and your heels are suspended. Place your shoulders snugly underneath the pads. Start with your knees slightly bent (keep them this way throughout the range of motion) and your heels dropped toward the floor below the level of the platform. Flex your calves to extend your ankles as high as possible. Squeeze your calves for 1-2 counts at the top, then lower back to the start position, feeling a stretch at the bottom.

Seated Calf Raise

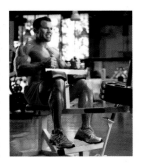

Sit on the seat and adjust the pads so they fit snugly on your lower thighs. Place the balls of your feet and toes on the platform so your heels are suspended. Release the safety catch and begin with your heels below the level of the platform so you feel a stretch in your calves. Extend your ankles to push the pads up as high as you can — you should be almost on your tiptoes at the top. Squeeze your calves, then lower back down.

Donkey Calf Raise

Step into a donkey calf raise machine and place the balls of your feet on the foot platform with your upper glutes/lower back secured under the pad provided. Allow your forearms to rest on the arm pad and grasp the handles. Press up onto your toes by contracting your calves, squeeze the contraction and lower your heels toward the floor as low as possible.

Smith Machine Calf Raise

Stand inside a Smith machine with the balls of your feet on a short platform. With the bar across your upper traps, let your heels travel down toward the floor for a good stretch, then press up onto your toes as high as possible.

Dumbbell Seated Calf Raise

Sit on the end of a flat bench or seat and place the balls of your feet on a raised surface (like a wood block) so that your heels are suspended. Place a pair of relatively heavy dumbbells on your lower quads, just above your knees, and begin with your heels below the level of the platform so you feel a stretch in your calves. Extend your ankles to push the dumbbells up as high as you can up onto on your tiptoes. Squeeze your calves, then lower back down.

SHOULDERS/TRAPS

Barbell Overhead Press

Sit on an upright bench or low-back seat with a barbell racked overhead. Grasp the bar just outside shoulder width, lift it off the rack (preferably with the help of a spotter) and begin with it overhead, arms extended. Slowly lower the bar in front of your face until it reaches about chin level, then explosively press it back up without locking out your elbows.

Dumbbell Overhead Press

Sit on an upright bench or low-back seat and hold a set of dumbbells at shoulder level, elbows and wrists stacked. Press the weights simultaneously up and in over your head until the dumbbells nearly touch, then reverse the motion to return to the start.

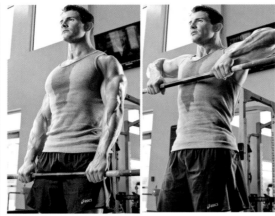

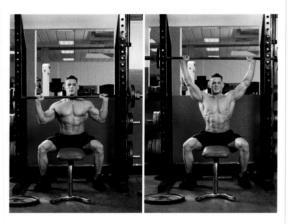

Smith Machine Overhead Press

Sit on a low-back seat or bench placed inside the machine with your feet flat on the floor. Grasp the bar with a wide, palms-forward grip. Keep your head straight and eyes forward. Rotate the bar to unrack it and hold it at shoulder level. Powerfully press the bar directly overhead, squeezing your shoulders at the top. Slowly lower to the start position and repeat.

Arnold Press

Sit on a low back seat holding a pair of dumbbells. Start with your elbows bent in front of you so that the dumbbells are at chin level and your palms and forearms face you, not forward. Press the dumbbells up overhead while simultaneously rotating your forearms until they face forward at the top of the movement. Slowly lower the weights back to the start position.

Upright Row

Stand holding a barbell in front of you with a shoulder-width grip and your arms extended down. Lift the bar straight up along your body by bending your elbows and contracting your delts until it reaches chest level. Hold the contraction for a count, then slowly lower the bar to full elbow extension.

Smith Machine Upright Row

Stand in a Smith machine holding the bar in front of your thighs with a shoulder-width grip, arms extended. Lift the bar straight up along your body by bending your elbows and contracting your delts until it reaches upper-chest level. Hold the contraction, then slowly lower the bar to full extension.

Dumbbell Lateral Raise

Stand holding a pair of relatively light dumbbells at your sides, arms extended. Lift the weights straight out to your sides in an arc until your arms are parallel to the floor. Hold the contraction for a count, then slowly lower the dumbbells back to your sides.

Machine Lateral Raise

Sit on the seat of a lateral raise machine so that your shoulders line up with the machine's axes of rotation. Depending on the type of machine, either grasp the handles with your hands or place your elbows on the pads with your upper arms pointed toward the floor. Contract your delts to lift your arms in an arc out to your sides until your upper arms are parallel with the floor. Pause, then slowly lower to the start position.

Dumbbell Front Raise

Hold two dumbbells in front of your thighs with your arms extended. The movement can be performed using either both arms simultaneously or one at a time. If you do single-arm reps, raise one dumbbell outward in front of you, keeping your elbow extended but not locked out, until your arm is about parallel to the floor. Lower the weight back to the start position under control, then do a rep with the opposite arm. Alternate arms until you complete your desired number of reps.

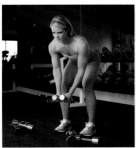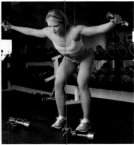

Bent-Over Lateral Raise

Hold a pair of dumbbells and lean forward at the waist so your torso is nearly parallel to the floor. Let your arms hang straight down, elbows extended and palms facing in; keep your chest up and back flat to avoid injury. Simultaneously lift the dumbbells in an arc out to your sides until your arms are roughly parallel to the floor. (Keep your elbows relatively straight; bending them excessively takes tension off your rear delts.) Lower the weights under control back to the start position; don't simply let them drop.

Cable Front Raise

Stand facing away from the weight stack of a low-pulley cable with a straight bar attached. Using an overhand grip, grasp the bar with both hands with the cable running between your legs. Pull the bar up and out in front of you until your arms are parallel to the floor. Squeeze for a count, then slowly lower to the start position without letting the weight rest on the stack between reps.

Reverse Pec-Deck Flye

Sit backward at a pec deck machine and grasp the handles in front of you with a neutral grip (palms facing each other). Keep your abs tight and your chest up. Flex your rear delts, keeping a slight bend in your elbows, to pull the handles back until your upper arms are just past perpendicular to your torso. Hold briefly, then return to the start position.

Barbell Shrug

Hold a barbell at arms' length in front of your thighs. Keeping your elbows extended, simply elevate ("shrug") your shoulders as high as you can — straight up and down, not backward or forward — and squeeze at the top. Lower back to the start position, depressing your shoulders, then repeat for reps.

Dumbbell Shrug

Stand erect with soft knees and hold a set of dumbbells at the outside of your thighs. Slowly contract through your traps to pull your shoulders toward your ears. Hold for a second at the top, then return to the start.

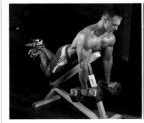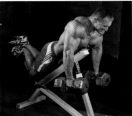

Incline Dumbbell Shrug

Lie facedown on an incline bench set at a 35–40-degree angle. With your chest flush against the bench and your knees bent and on the seat, hold a dumbbell in each hand with a neutral (palms facing in) grip, arms hanging straight down. Shrug your shoulders as high as possible, squeeze your traps for a count or two, then slowly lower the dumbbells straight down to the start position.

Smith Machine Behind-the-Back Shrug

Stand directly in front of the bar with your feet spaced about shoulder-width apart. Grasp the bar with an overhand grip and your hands just outside your hips. Rotate the bar to unrack it. Keeping your arms straight, chest up and eyes facing forward, shrug your shoulders upward, bringing your delts toward your ears. Hold the peak contraction and squeeze for a count before lowing the bar to the start position. Repeat for reps.

TRICEPS

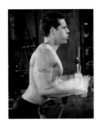

Triceps Pushdown

Stand facing a cable stack and attach a straight-bar, EZ-bar, V-bar or rope handle to a high-pulley cable. Grasp the attachment with both hands and begin with your elbows tight at your sides and your forearms just shy of parallel to the floor. Keeping your elbows in, extend your arms until they're straight, squeezing your triceps at the bottom of the rep.

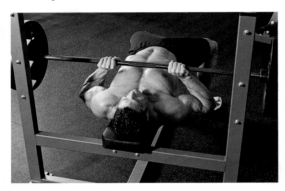

Close-Grip Bench Press

Position yourself as you would when benching, but grasp the bar (loaded with a lighter weight than you'd use for wide-grip benching) with your hands 6–12 inches apart. Lower the bar to your mid-to-lower chest, then press it back up explosively, keeping your elbows as close to your sides as possible.

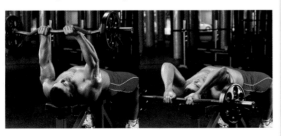

Lying Barbell Triceps Extension

Lie faceup on a flat bench, holding a weighted EZ-bar at arm's length over your face. Keeping your elbows pulled in, slowly lower the bar toward the top of your head. Before it touches, pause, then contract your triceps to press back up to the start position.

Cable Overhead Extension

Attach a rope to a high pulley on a cable apparatus. Stand facing away from the stack, grasp the rope near the knots and hold the attachment behind your head. Bend forward at your waist so your torso is at approximately a 45-degree angle to the floor and start the move with your elbows bent less than 90 degrees and your hands still behind your head. Keeping your elbows pressed together, extend your arms so your hands move forward in front of your head. Squeeze your triceps at full elbow extension by turning your palms out, then return to the start position.

Dumbbell Lying Triceps Extension

Lie faceup on a flat bench and hold a pair of dumbbells at arms' length straight above you. Keeping your elbows pulled together, lower the dumbbells slowly toward your forehead. When your elbows reach slightly beyond 90 degrees, press the weights back up to the start position by contracting your triceps.

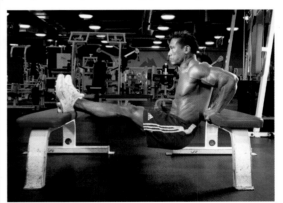

Bench Dip

Place two benches a few feet apart and parallel to each other. Sit on the middle of one bench facing the other. Place your hands just outside your hips on the bench, cupping the bench with your fingers. Place your heels on the opposite bench, pressing yourself upward so your body forms an "L" in the top position. Slowly lower your glutes toward the floor until your arms form 90-degree angles. Pause, then forcefully press yourself back up to the start position. This exercise can also be done with additional weight by having a partner place one or more weight plates on your lap at the beginning of the set.